Register &
Access

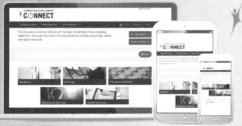

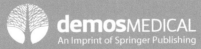

Interventional Pain
Procedures

Interventional Pain Procedures

Handbook and Video Guide

Michael Sabia, MD

Division Head Pain Management
Pain Medicine Fellowship Director
Assistant Professor of Anesthesiology
Cooper Medical School of Rowan University
Department of Anesthesiology
Division of Pain Management
Voorhees, New Jersey

Rajat Mathur, MD

Pain Management Specialist
Department of Rehabilitation Medicine
Division of Pain Management
MedStar Georgetown University School of Medicine
Washington, DC

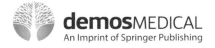

demosMEDICAL
An Imprint of Springer Publishing

Visit our website at www.springerpub.com

ISBN: 9781620701027
ebook ISBN: 9781617052798

Acquisitions Editor: Beth Barry
Compositor: diacriTech

Medicine is an ever-changing science. Research and clinical experience are continually expanding our knowledge, in particular our understanding of proper treatment and drug therapy. The authors, editors, and publisher have made every effort to ensure that all information in this book is in accordance with the state of knowledge at the time of production of the book. Nevertheless, the authors, editors, and publisher are not responsible for errors or omissions or for any consequences from application of the information in this book and make no warranty, expressed or implied, with respect to the contents of the publication. Every reader should examine carefully the package inserts accompanying each drug and should carefully check whether the dosage schedules mentioned therein or the contraindications stated by the manufacturer differ from the statements made in this book. Such examination is particularly important with drugs that are either rarely used or have been newly released on the market.

Library of Congress Cataloging-in-Publication Data
Names: Sabia, Michael, author. | Mathur, Rajat, author.
Title: Interventional pain procedures : handbook and video guide / Michael
    Sabia, Rajat Mathur.
Description: New York : Springer Publishing Company, [2018]
Identifiers: LCCN 2018000374| ISBN 9781620701027 | ISBN 9781617052798 (e-book)
Subjects: | MESH: Pain Management—methods | Spine—surgery | Spinal Cord
    Stimulation | Autonomic Nerve Block—methods | Radiography, Interventional
    | Handbooks
Classification: LCC RD768 | NLM WL 39 | DDC 617.4/71—dc23
LC record available at https://lccn.loc.gov/2018000374

Contact us to receive discount rates on bulk purchases.
We can also customize our books to meet your needs.
For more information please contact: sales@springerpub.com

Printed in the United States of America.
21 22 23 24 / 6 5 4 3

To my mom and dad, your love and guidance ignited a fire inside of me which allows me to give my all everyday. Your presence alone fuels my hunger to improve the quality of care I render to patients on a daily basis. I'm forever grateful for the life you've provided for me. Thank you for believing in me and supporting me throughout this lifetime journey.

To my children, Sebastian and Milana, I promise to love and care for you until the end of time. Hard work, determination, and being regimented are the key ingredients to success.

To the staff at Cooper University Hospital and the Voorhees Surgery Center. I am eternally thankful for the excellent training I've received. Being around a group of such talented and dynamic healthcare providers helped nurture my passion for healing pain and suffering.

Michael Sabia

To my wife, thank you for your understanding and unconditional love. You make me and everyone you come across a better human being, I TRULY cannot imagine life without you.

To my mom and dad, I am who I am because of you both. Thank you for your trust, values, and most importantly love. My dreams would be impossible without you both!

To my sister, thank you for your trust and belief in me, especially during those times when I did not believe in myself!

To my son, your presence in my life brings me the kind of happiness that I did not know was possible. I am excited to be a part of your life and know you will make the world a better place.

To Dr. Michael Sabia, thank you for being my role model of what a physician should be and a wonderful mentor to me.

Rajat Mathur

Contents

List of Videos

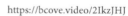

Preface

Image-guided interventions for pain management have evolved since being performed with palpation guidance. The utilization of fluoroscopic guided interventions for pain management has emerged in treating painful spinal conditions. During residency or fellowship, the trainee often has limited experience in standard of care and broad interventional pain management techniques. Although, there are a wide variety of excellent sources, there has been a lack of use of multimedia utilization in teaching interventional pain management techniques.

Our goal with this handbook is to provide a rapid and accurate reference for interventional pain management physicians, allow dynamic teaching of interventional procedures, and understanding and visualizing interventional techniques for commonly performed interventional pain management procedures. The handbook also describes etiology, physical examination techniques, and treatment plans of common painful conditions treated by an interventional pain management physician.

We would also like to thank Dr. Ramesh Mathur for the medical illustrations used in this text.

Michael Sabia
Rajat Mathur

Anatomy of the Spine and Spinal Cord for Pain Procedures

SPINE

The spine is made up of 33 individual bones stacked with ligaments and muscles connecting the bones together to maintain alignment. The vertebral column consists of 33 vertebrae (seven cervical; 12 thoracic; five lumbar; five sacral; four coccyx). C1 and C2 are atypical (Figure 1.1).

The main purpose of the spine is to support the trunk and protect the spinal cord. The spinal column provides the main support for your body, allowing you to stand upright, twist, and bend.

Primary curvatures are located in the thoracic and sacral regions, and secondary curvatures are located in the cervical and lumbar region. Abnormal curvatures of the vertebral column include the following:

- Kyphosis: abnormally increased thoracic curvature
- Lordosis: abnormally increased lumbar curvature
- Scoliosis: lateral deviation of the spine

Vertebra change in size and shape from cranial to caudal by getting larger and thicker. Typical vertebra consists of a body and a vertebral arch with several processes for articular and muscular attachments.

- The function of the vertebral body is to support weight. The vertebral body is bound together by intervertebral disks resulting in the formation of cartilaginous joints.
- The neural (vertebral) arch consists of paired pedicles bilaterally and paired laminae posteriorly. The neural arch forms the neural foramen with the vertebral body and protects the spinal cord and nerve root (Figure 1.2).

The vertebral arch is associated with five processes:

- Transverse processes project bilaterally from the junction of the lamina and pedicle. The transverse processes articulate with the rib tubercles from T1 to T10.

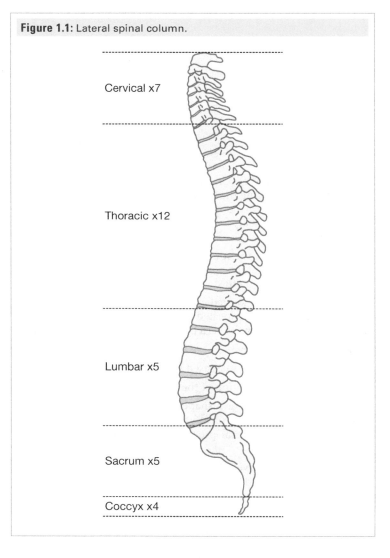

Figure 1.1: Lateral spinal column.

Cervical x7

Thoracic x12

Lumbar x5

Sacrum x5

Coccyx x4

- Spinous processes are located from C3 to C7, T1 to T12, and L1 to L5, and project posteriorly from the junction of the two laminae of the vertebral arch.

- Articular processes (zygapophyses) are two superior and two inferior projections of the vertebrae that serve the purpose of

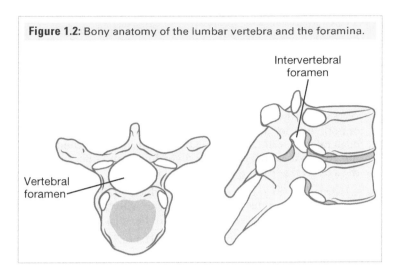

Figure 1.2: Bony anatomy of the lumbar vertebra and the foramina.

fitting an adjacent vertebra, forming a region of contact referred to as articular facet. The superior processes project upward from the lower vertebra, and their articular surfaces are directed backward. The inferior processes project downward from the higher vertebra, and their articular surfaces are directed forward and outward.

- Mammillary processes are small apophysis or tubercles on the dorsal margin of the superior articular process of each lumbar vertebra and usually the 12th thoracic vertebra.

- Accessory processes are small apophysis at the posterior part of the base of transverse process of each lumbar vertebra.

Foraminas of the vertebra:

- Transverse foramina are small foramina usually seen in C1 to C6 vertebral bodies. They contain vertebral arteries as well as autonomic nerves and small veins.

- Intervertebral foramina, also known as neural foramina, is a foramina between the inferior and superior surface of the pedicles of adjacent vertebrae. It allows passage of the spinal nerves and accompanying vessels as they exit the vertebral canal.

- Vertebral foramina are formed by vertebral bodies and arches. The vertebral foraminas form the canal and transmit the spinal cord with its meningeal coverings, nerve roots, and vessels.

Special characteristics of the spine:

- Cervical vertebra differs from the thoracic and lumbar vertebra because they have smaller bodies, foramen for vertebral arteries, and a larger vertebral canal to house the cervical spinal cord enlargement.

- C1 Atlas supports the skull, and is the widest of the cervical vertebrae. It has no body and no spinous process but consists of both anterior and posterior arches and transverse processes bilaterally. Superiorly, it articulates with the occipital condyles of the skull to form the atlanto-occipital joints, and inferiorly with the axis (C2) to form the atlantoaxial joints.

- C2 Axis has an odontoid process, which projects superiorly from the body of the axis and articulates with the anterior arch of the atlas, allowing a pivot motion for the atlas.

- C2–C6 are similarly shaped cervical vertebrae which have short bifid spinous process and transverse processes with a transverse foramina for the vertebral vessels.

- C7 is also known as vertebra prominens. It has a long spinous process that is horizontal and forms a visible protrusion due to its thickness.

- Thoracic vertebrae have costal facets (superior, transverse, and inferior). The superior costal facet is a site where the rib forms a joint with the top of a vertebra. The transverse costal facet is a site where a rib forms a joint with the transverse process of the thoracic vertebra. The inferior costal facet is a site where a rib forms a joint with the inferior aspect of the body of a thoracic vertebra.

- Lumbar vertebrae are distinguished by their large bodies and are designed to carry most of the body's weight. The body of L5 is the largest body of the vertebrae. They do not have costal facets.

- Sacrum is a fused, large triangular-shaped bone. It is located behind the bones forming the pelvis. It contains four foramina bilaterally to form the exit of the ventral and dorsal roots of the first four sacral nerves. The superior and lateral part of the sacrum is called the sacral ala, which is formed by the fused transverse processes and fused costal processes of the first sacral vertebra. The sacral hiatus is a normally occurring gap at the lower end of the sacrum, exposing the vertebral canal. It is formed by the failure of the laminae S5 to fuse. When performing a caudal epidural, the sacral hiatus is entered.

- Coccyx is formed by the union of four coccygeal vertebrae.

Intervertebral disks:

- The annulus fibrosus is a shock absorber as it is the tough collagenous circular exterior of the intervertebral disc that surrounds and maintains the integrity of the nucleus pulposus.
- Nucleus pulposus is in the central portion of the intervertebral disk and may herniate through the annulus fibrosis, causing impingement of the roots of the spinal nerves. The primary function of the nucleus pulposus is for shock absorption.

Ligaments of the spine:

- Anterior longitudinal ligament is a long, thick ligament that traverses the entire length of the spinal canal and helps provide stability to the spinal column. It is situated anteriorly to the spinal cord in the spinal column, and it helps limit flexion and prevent overextension. It also resists the gravitational pull.
- Posterior longitudinal ligament allows interconnection of the vertebral bodies and intervertebral disks which supports the posterior aspect of the spine. The main function is to limit flexion of the spine. Occasionally, this ligament is a pain generator causing axial low back pain.
- Ligamentum flavum is a short but thick ligament that connects the laminae of vertebrae from C2 to S1. In the neck region, the ligament is thin, broad, and long. It is thick in the thoracic region but thickest in the lumbar region. The ligament may hypertrophy causing spinal stenosis because it lies in the posterior portion of the spinal column. It may also calcify causing it to be difficult to pierce during a spinal injection.
- Ligamentum nuchae is located between the muscles on both sides of the posterior aspect of the neck. It is formed by thickened supraspinous ligaments that extend from C7 vertebra to the occipital protuberance. It is attached from the posterior tubercle of the atlas and to the spinous processes of the cervical vertebrae (Figure 1.3).

Biomechanics of the spine:

- Thoracolumbar spine:
    1. Upper thoracic zone (T1–T8) is rigid due to the rib cage which provides protection and stability.
    2. Transition zone (T9–L2) is the transition between the rigid and kyphotic region and the flexible lumbar spine. This region is where more injuries occur.

Figure 1.3: Ligaments of the spine.

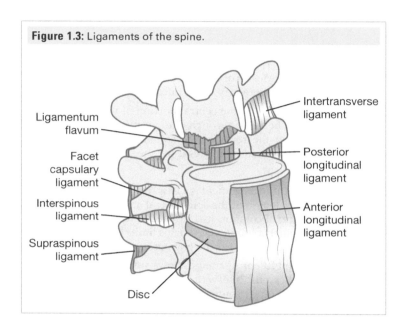

Ligamentum flavum

Facet capsulary ligament

Interspinous ligament

Supraspinous ligament

Disc

Intertransverse ligament

Posterior longitudinal ligament

Anterior longitudinal ligament

3. L3 Sacrum zone is flexible. This region is where axial loading injuries occur.

Three-column model of Denis:

1. Model is used to predict soft tissue injury from bone injury. It contains anterior column, middle column, and posterior column.

   a. Anterior column elements: vertebral bodies, intervertebral discs, rami communicantes, lumbar sympathetic chain

   b. Middle column elements: pedicles, neural foramina and contents, central canal and contents

   c. Posterior column elements: facet joint, lamina, pars interarticularis, facet articular processes, paraspinous muscles, spinous process, SI joint (Figures 1.4 and 1.5)

   d. Intact spinal stability requires two intact columns. Instability is the result of two-third column disruption. For example, a burst fracture is always unstable because at least the anterior and middle column integrity is disrupted

Figure 1.4: A schematic of the three-column model of Denis.

3-Column Model of Denis

Anterior column   Middle column   Posterior column

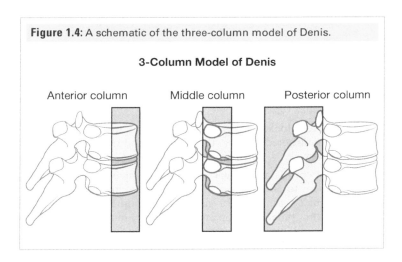

Figure 1.5: X-ray of the anterior middle and posterior columns.

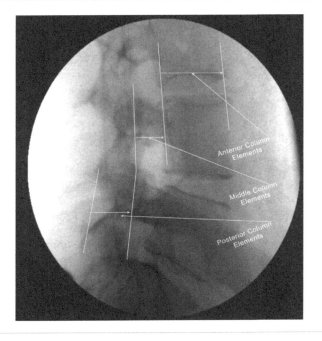

SPINAL CORD

The spinal cord lies within the subarachnoid space and extends from the foramen magnum where it continues from the medulla oblongata at the spinomedullary junction to the level of the first or second lumbar vertebra.

The filum terminale is an extension of the pia mater that extends from the conus medullaris to the dural sac and from the dural sac to the coccyx.

The spinal cord is an elongated and nearly cylindrical structure, and is 40 cm to 50 cm long and 1 cm to 1.5 cm in diameter. In length, a male's spinal cord averages 45 cm and 42 cm in females. In adults, the spinal cord usually ends at the junction between the first and second lumbar vertebra. Variations include as high as T12 and as low as L3.

There are three membranes called the meninges, which surround and protect the spinal cord. The cerebrospinal fluid (CSF) is a clear body fluid and it circulates between the meninges, brain, and spinal cord. Its function is to protect the central nervous system. The three meninges are the following:

- The dura mater is made of strong connective tissue and is a gray outer layer of the spinal cord and nerve roots.

- The arachnoid membrane comes in direct contact with the dura mater and is separated from the pia mater by a CSF-filled space called the subarachnoid space. It contains arteries and veins.

- The pia mater is the innermost and highly vascular membrane allowing blood to go to the spinal cord and nerve roots.

EPIDURAL SPACE

The epidural space is outside the dura mater and contains fat, lymphatics, areolar tissue, spinal nerve roots, and the internal vertebral venous plexus (Batson's venous plexus). It extends from the foramen magnum to the sacral hiatus. Identification of the epidural space when delivering epidural medication involves the measurement of loss of resistance using glass or plastic syringes. This is crucial and technically demanding. The accuracy in the location of the epidural needle in space determines the functionality of the administration of medicine into the epidural space. In the cervical region, the loss of resistance is poorly appreciated since the ligamentum flavum is thin and nonexistent in some patients. The distance from ligamentum flavum to dura is approximately 1.5 mm to 2 mm at C7, and increased to 3 mm to 4 mm with neck flexion. The epidural space shows a slight increase in diameter the further caudad you go. Thoracic epidural space measures approximately 2 mm to 4 mm, lumbar epidural space measures approximately 4 mm to 6 mm. In the lumbar region, it is advised to enter below the L2 level to avoid the spinal cord (Table 1.1; Figure 1.6).

One of the most reliable methods in identifying the space depends on loss of the residence technique. This method involves the use

TABLE 1.1: EPIDURAL SPACE BOUNDARIES

Anteriorly	Posterior longitudinal ligament, vertebral discs, and bodies
Posteriorly	Ligamentum flavum, capsule of facet joints, and laminae
Laterally	Pedicles and intervertebral foramina
Superiorly	Fusion of the spinal and periosteal layers of dura mater at the foramen magnum
Inferiorly	Sacrococcygeal membranes

Figure 1.6: Transverse section of the lumbar vertebra.

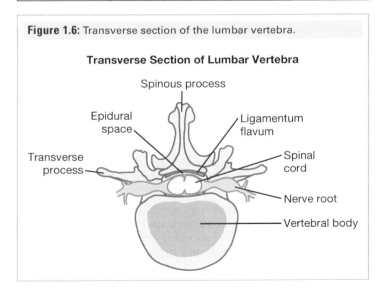

Transverse Section of Lumbar Vertebra

Spinous process

Epidural space

Ligamentum flavum

Transverse process

Spinal cord

Nerve root

Vertebral body

of liquid such as saline or air to achieve "the loss." This technique involves continuous or intermittent pressure on the piston of an epidural glass or plastic syringe attached to the epidural needle, allowing the piston to move into the barrel. As the needle is placed into the ligamentum flavum and held steady by the nondominant hand, the dominant hand holds the syringe. Steady pressure is applied to the plunger to compress the air bubble present in the syringe. The needle is advanced slowly and steadily until the loss of resistance is noted.

Epidural space may also be identified by a hanging drop technique that involves the placement of the needle into the ligamentum flavum. Next, the Tuohy needle shaft is filled with a few drops of preservative-free normal saline so a visible drop is noticed at the hub of the needle. A slow and steady pressure is applied to advance the needle until the hanging drop gets sucked in due to the subatmospheric pressure present in the epidural space.

SPINAL NERVES

There are thirty-one pairs of spinal nerves (eight cervical, 12 thoracic, five lumbar, five sacral, and one coccygeal).

Nerves arising directly from the spinal cord are called spinal nerves or nerve roots. The spinal nerves branch off the spinal cord and pass out through a hole in each of the vertebra called the foramen. Two consecutive rows of nerve roots emerge from both sides of the spinal cord. The dorsal root ganglia (DRG) lives in the lateral recesses bilaterally. Spinal nerves carry information to and from different segments in the spinal cord. There are 31 pairs of spinal nerves that branch off from the spinal cord. In the cervical region of the spinal cord, the spinal nerves exit above the vertebrae. The C8 spinal nerve exits the vertebra below the C7 vertebra. Starting with the first thoracic vertebra downward, all spinal nerves exit below their associated numbered vertebrae.

The C1 nerve passes between the atlas and the skull; all other spinal nerves exit the vertebral canal via the intervertebral canal or sacral foramina.

1. The C1–C3 spinal nerves are primarily responsible for transmission of pain signals from the neck to the head. The ventral ramus of the C1 spinal nerve innervates the short muscles of the suboccipital triangle and atlanto-occipital joint.

2. The C1, C2, and C3 sinuvertebral branches innervate the dura mater over the clivus in the posterior cranial fossa.

3. The ventral ramus of C2 spinal nerve innervates the sternocleidomastoid and the trapezius muscles, as well as the lateral atlantoaxial joint.

4. The dorsal ramus of C2 innervates the splenius capitis and semispinalis capitis, and its medial branch innervates the occipital area (greater occipital nerve).

5. The C3 ventral ramus innervates the prevertebral musculature.

6. The C3 dorsal ramus (lesser occipital nerve) innervates the posterior cervical musculature, splenius capitis, cervicis, longissimus capitis, semispinalis, cervicis, and multifidus, and its superficial medial branch innervates the C2–C3 zygapophyseal joint (third occipital nerve).

7. The C3 sinuvertebral branch innervates the C2–C3 intervertebral disc.

The spinal nerve is formed by the fusion of posterior and anterior roots within the intervertebral foramen.

There are four main groups of spinal nerves, which exit from different levels of the spinal cord.

- Cervical nerves: innervate the neck region, allow movement and feeling to the arms, neck, and upper trunk. The cervical nerves also control breathing.

- Thoracic nerves: innervate the upper back region, trunk, and abdomen.

- Lumbar and sacral nerves: innervate the lower back, legs, the bowel and bladder, and the sexual organs.

C-Arm Overview

The main purpose of the fluoroscope is to generate a controllable beam of x-rays which is directed through the tissue to produce an image. The benefits of the C-arm fluoroscope are that it has a compact design and can be easily maneuvered. The C-arm works in conjunction with a table that is designed for C-arms.

C-arm has four main components:

- The image intensifier allows low-intensity x-rays to be amplified, resulting in decreased radiation exposure to patient and enabling the practitioner to easily view the image.

- The x-ray source is where the power to penetrate the body comes from, allowing greater flexibility for imaging while reducing the exposure times. This allows easier imaging on obese patients and less risk for error. It consists of an input window, input phosphor, photocathode, vacuum and electron optics, output phosphor, and output window.

- The imaging system unit can perform a variety of movements that allow for use in a variety of procedures. The C-arm has a range of movements including rotation, tilts, raise, lower, and extension.

- The workstation on the C-arm allows operation of the C-arm including exposure switch, controls of radiographic settings, fluoroscopic settings, hard and optical disks, image quality enhancement software, noise reduction, zoom control, save and swapping images, and so forth.

RADIATION SAFETY

There are approximately seven to 10 million interventional pain procedures performed annually in the United States, with 50% of these being performed under fluoroscopy. Fluoroscopy is used for the major purpose of ensuring proper needle placement and visualization of the delivery of the injectate. It is also utilized to decrease possible side effects and enhance the safety of the patient. Fluoroscopy use does cause radiation exposure to patients, physicians, and other personnel. Overuse of the fluoroscope may result in injuries to skin, muscle, the lens of the eye, and may result in injury to internal organs as well.

Radiation exposure during fluoroscopy is directly proportional to the length of time the unit is activated by the foot pedal or image switch. Unlike regular x-ray units, fluoroscopic units do not have an automatic timer to terminate the exposure after it is activated. Instead, activation of the x-ray switch determines the length of the exposure which ceases only after the switch is released. Thus, cognizance of beam on time is extremely important to fluoroscopy safety.

Biologic Effects of X-Rays

There are two major biological effects of radiation exposure: nonstochastic and stochastic.

- Nonstochastic effects are also referred to as deterministic or tissue and organ effects and are specific to each exposed individual. If an individual is exposed to low-dose radiation once or a few times, the nonstochastic effects will not be apparent. However, interventional pain physicians and other involved personnel are chronically exposed to low-dose radiation. Cataracts, erythema, epilation, and even death are examples of nonstochastic effects.

- Stochastic effects are those which occur by chance and are more difficult to identify. The stochastic effect is one in which the probability of the effect increases with the radiation dose rather than the severity. The main stochastic effects are cancer and genetic defects. There is no known existing threshold for stochastic effects. For these reasons, the stochastic effect is also called the linear or zero-threshold dose-response effect. Since there is no evidence of a lower threshold for the appearance of stochastic effects, the sensible course of action is to ensure that all radiation exposure follow the principle **ALARA (as low as reasonably achievable)**. It is recommended that interventional pain physicians use ALARA as a work principle, a mindset, and teach it as a culture of professional excellence.

Figure 2.1: Suboptimal and optimal practice to reduce radiation exposure.

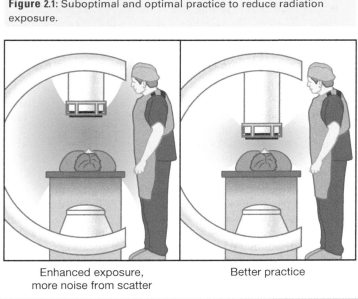

Enhanced exposure,   Better practice
more noise from scatter

Operator exposure profile (Figure 2.1):

- No portion of the operator's body should be in the primary beam during imaging. Due to this, the majority of the radiation dose received by the operator is due to scattered radiation from the patient. Following interaction with the patient, radiation is scattered more or less uniformly in all directions.

- It is vital to note that the patient does not uniformly emit this scattered radiation because some of the scattered radiation is absorbed or reduced in intensity by passing through the patient. The intensity of scatter decreases with increasing distance from the patient. Consequently, scatter radiation is highest near its source (i.e., the x-ray beam entry point on the patient). Since radiation is scattered in the forward direction, it is subjected to the most tissue attenuation, radiation levels are significantly lower on the contralateral side than the x-ray tube side.

- Highest scatter radiation levels most often occur where the operator stands. Radiation levels increase with decreasing distance from the point of x-ray entry. In general, an operator positioned 3 ft from the x-ray beam entrance area will receive .1% of the patient's exposure at skin entrance. Staff members positioned further away receive much less exposure due to inverse square law effects. In almost all cases, the tableside operator will receive the highest occupational radiation exposure during the fluoroscopic procedure. Tableside fluoroscopy operators receive among the highest occupational radiation exposures within the health system.

Radiation quantities and units:

- The quantity that is used to assess the energy deposited in tissues from radiation is the absorbed dose. In the current International System of Units, the unit of absorbed dose is the joule/kilogram with the special name of gray (Gy). 1 Gy = 100 rad. An absorbed dose of 1 Gy is 100 times the magnitude of the older unit of absorbed dose, the rad. Thus, a dose rate to skin of .02 Gy/min is equivalent to 2 rad/min.

- The greatest single source of man-made radiation exposure to the average person in the United States comes from medical irradiation. Medical doses range from a few millirads for a chest x-ray to thousands of rads in the treatment of cancer.

- Fluoroscopic procedures (particularly prolonged interventional procedures) may involve high patient radiation doses. The radiation dose depends on the type of examination, the patient size, the equipment, the technique, and many other factors. The performance of the fluoroscopy system with respect to radiation dose is best characterized by the receptor entrance exposure and skin entrance exposure rates, which should be assessed at regular intervals.

- The two major risks associated with fluoroscopy are radiation-induced injuries to the skin and underlying tissues ("burns") and the small possibility of developing a radiation-induced cancer some time later in life.

- When an individual has a medical need, the benefit of an x-ray procedure far exceeds the small cancer risk associated with the procedure. However, even when medically necessary, it is advisable to use the lowest possible exposure.

Guidelines for occupational exposure:

- All procedure room personnel should wear a protective lead apron and thyroid shield (minimum .5 mm lead equivalency). A good practitioner will alert everyone in the room that he or she is about to start fluoroscopy use. If the walls of the procedure room are adjacent to the waiting room, wall shielding should be considered.

- Individuals who are in the procedure suite on a daily basis are recommended to wear dosimetry badges. Dosimetry badges are radiation detection clips that are used to measure cumulative radiation exposure. To determine efficacy of the lead apron and overall exposure, two badges may be worn, one inside the lead apron and one outside the lead apron. These badges are analyzed every 30 days to allow monitoring of cumulative radiation exposure. Leaded eyeglasses may also be used to provide a barrier to eye exposure and decrease the incidence of the theoretical cataract risk from radiation exposure. Lead glass screens may also be used in between the operator and the x-ray source to reduce the direct and radiation scatter.

- Current exposure to individuals who work with radiation is set to the upper effective dose equivalent of 50 mSv (5 rem/y) and a cumulative dose should not exceed to 10 mSv (1 rem) times the age of the individual.

- Symptoms of radiation injury often present in a delayed fashion, and are not immediately apparent. Also, fluoroscopy-induced injuries are underreported, thus the actual extent of the problem is unknown.

Radiographic Contrast Agents

To ensure accurate and precise needle placement when performing interventional pain management injections under fluoroscopic guidance, it is recommended that contrast dye is used. Current contrast agents have an iodine base which may be bound to an organic compound or an ionic compound. Ionic compounds generally have a higher osmolality and more side effects. Anaphylactoid reactions, seizures, and anaphylactic reactions have been reported with the use of contrast media. Nonionic water-soluble contrast agents are most commonly used in current practice. Some examples of these nonionic contrast agents are iohexol (Omnipaque 350), which is the only agent approved from intrathecal administration; iopamidol (Isovue 370); iopromide (Ultravist 370); ioxilan (Oxilan 350); and iodixanol (Visipaque 320).

Spread of nonionic contrast agents in the epidural space is known as an epidurogram. Interpretation of an epidurogram is an important skill that allows an interventional pain physician to perform safe practice for delivery of epidural medications (e.g., steroids, local anesthetics) or blood (blood patch) in the cervical, thoracic, and lumbar spine. To avoid dural sac compression, spinal cord compression, and loculation of contrast dye, one should use as little dye as possible to perform and interpret an epidurogram.

Other important contrast dye patterns that can occur with spinal injections are intrathecal, subdural, intravascular, intraneuronal, intradiscal, and intra-articular. It is recommended that contrast dye be injected under live/real-time fluoroscopy for all transforaminal epidural steroid injections to observe for any radicular artery/feeder vessel uptake. Injection of particulate steroids into these vascular structures can lead to a devastating spinal cord infarct progressing to paraplegia, tetraplegia, or quadriplegia. Triamcinolone and depo-methylprednisolone are the common particulate steroids that are used in most pain practices today. Dexamethasone is the only steroid most likely free of particulate matter available for epidural injections.

Contrast-induced nephropathy is a rare complication that occurs when performing spinal injections, mostly because the total volume/concentration/dose of dye is small (relative to the amount used in arteriograms).

NEEDLE ANATOMY AND TECHNIQUES

Spinal needles with a Quincke point (Figure 2.2):

- This type of spinal needle has many advantages including accurate application and flexibility. The needle is advanced easily and due to the stylet, a biopsy effect is prevented. This is due to the Quincke tip with a double bevel which enables atraumatic punctures as it is advanced. This minimizes adverse events such as excessive bleeding.

- This type of needle is manufactured from steel that is high quality and it also has a thin-walled cannula. This allows the surface of the needle to be smooth, allowing an atraumatic puncture of tissue.

- In addition to the ergonomic design to allow easy manipulation, the needle hub is transparent, which allows quick detection of heme of cerebrospinal fluid backflow. This feature allows precise positioning of the needle tip.

- These needles are sterilized by ethylene oxide and are single patient use. They have a shelf life of approximately 5 years.

Figure 2.2: A Quincke needle.

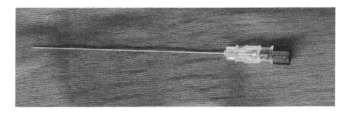

Figure 2.3: A modified Tuohy needle.

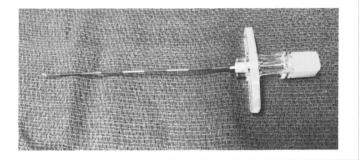

Tuohy needle (Figure 2.3):

- The Tuohy is a blunt hypodermic needle that is slightly curved at the end and is the most common needle for delivery of medications into the epidural space.

- The stylet has a notch that is used to indicate the bevel orientation. The needle and stylet fit together to give a smooth bevel surface and thus minimize the coring of the skin and other subcutaneous tissues.

- The needles are also sterilized by ethylene oxide and are single patient use. They have a shelf life of approximately 5 years.

Extension tubing:

- After the needle tip is placed in the final position, a luer-lock extension tubing is recommended to minimize needle tip movement or needle displacement. An extension tubing is also utilized to increase the distance of the physician's hand and the x-ray beam.

NONSTEROIDAL ANTI-INFLAMMATORIES

Nonsteroidal anti-inflammatory drugs (NSAIDs) decrease inflammation thus decreasing joint and musculoskeletal pain. The mechanism of action is by inhibition of the cyclooxygenase (COX) enzyme, leading to inhibition of prostaglandin synthesis. In general, use NSAIDs with caution in patients with renal and/or hepatic failure, gastrointestinal (GI) disease, or in patients receiving concurrent anticoagulation. Consider adding proton pump inhibitors or H_2 blockers in patients with high risk for developing upper GI bleeding associated with NSAIDs usage.

NSAID	DOSAGES	CONSIDERATIONS
Ibuprofen (Motrin)	400, 600, 800 mg	Maximum 2,400–3,200 mg/d
Sulindac (Clinoril)	150, 200 mg BID	Maximum 400 mg/d Safest NSAID for use in patients with renal problems.
Celecoxib (Celebrex)	100–200 mg daily or BID dose	Maximum 400 mg/d Preferred in patients at risk for GI side effects, GI ulcers, gastritis, or warfarin treatment Increased cardiovascular side effects of myocardial infarction and stroke

(continued)

NSAID	DOSAGES	CONSIDERATIONS
Naproxen (Naprosyn)	250, 375, 500 mg BID–TID dosing	Maximum 1,250 mg/d
Diclofenac (Voltaren)	50, 75 mg	Also comes in 1% gel
Diclofenac/ misoprostol (Arthrotec)	50/.2, 75/.2	
Etodolac (Lodine)	200–600 mg	
Indomethacin (Indocin)	25–50 mg 75 ER	
Oxaprozin (Daypro)	600 mg	Maximum 1,800 mg/d
Nabumetone (Relafen)	500–750 mg BID	Maximum 1,500 mg/d

GI, gastrointestinal; NSAID, nonsteroidal anti-inflammatory drug.

OPIOIDS

Opioids act as agonists at specific opioid receptors that are normally activated by endogenous ligands called endorphins and G protein-coupled receptors located in the spinal cord and brain stem. Opioids impede calcium transport by voltage-gated calcium channels. Opioids also impede release of acetylcholine, dopamine, norepinephrine, and substance P. Opioids produce analgesics activity by inhibiting the release of acetylcholine from nerve endings. Opioid-related side effects include constipation, nausea, and/or vomiting, drowsiness, delirium, and respiratory depression. Consider adding Colace and/or Senna for patients who are at high risk for developing opioid-induced constipation.

Constipation can also be treated with peripherally acting opioid receptor antagonists such as alvimopan.

Opioid-induced sedation or respiratory depression is secondary to μ-receptor activation. Opioid toxicity is treated with naloxone.

Opioid rotation should be considered if the current opioid is ineffective, there are adverse effects and/or toxicity of current opioid, or incomplete cross-tolerance. The opioid should be changed for another of equianalgesic potency which leads to a more favorable side-effect profile.

Opioid tolerance can be addressed by using N-methyl-D-aspartate (NMDA) antagonists, coadministration of NSAIDs, alpha-2-agonist, or initiation of opioid rotation.

Opioids are associated with many negative drug interactions and can be problematic in polypharmacy patients. Opioids, specifically methadone, are associated with decreased intermediate recall and learning. Chronic pain patients taking opioids have a lower employment rate than those not taking opioids. Opioids may aggravate depression and anxiety disorders in patients with chronic pain and have not been shown to improve either of these psychologic comorbidities in this patient population.

OPIOID	DOSAGES	CONSIDERATIONS
Acetaminophen with codeine (Tylenol #3)	APAP 300 mg with codeine 30–60 mg	Codeine is a low-potency opioid.
Fentanyl transdermal patch (Duragesic)	25, 50, 75, 100 mcg/hr	
Fentanyl transmucosal (Actiq)	200, 400, 600, 800, 1,200, 1,600 mcg	
Fentanyl transmucosal (Fentora)	100, 200, 400, 600, 800 mcg	
Fentanyl transmucosal (Subsys)	100, 200, 400, 600, 800 mcg spray	
Fentanyl nasal (Lazanda)	100, 400 mcg spray	

(*continued*)

(continued)

OPIOID	DOSAGES	CONSIDERATIONS
Hydrocodone with APAP (Vicodin)	5/300 mg 7.5/300 mg 10/300 mg	q4–6h PRN
Hydrocodone/ acetaminophen (Norco)	5/325 mg 7.5/325 mg	q4–6h PRN
Hydrocodone/ acetaminophen (Hycet)	10/325 mg 7.5/325/15 mL	q4–6h PRN
Hydrocodone (Hysingla ER)	20, 30, 40, 60, 80, 100, 120 mg PO QD	
Hydrocodone (Zohydro ER)	10, 15, 20, 30, 40, 50 mg QD	
Hydromorphone HCL (Dilaudid)	2 mg, 4 mg, and 8 mg tabs	High abuse potential 7x potent as morphine
Hydromorphone (Exalgo)	8, 12, 16, 32 mg	Long-acting
Methadone	5, 10 mg tabs	Antagonist for noncompetitive NMDA receptor
Morphine sulfate immediate release	15, 30, mg	High affinity for the μ-receptor
MS Contin extended release	15, 30, 60, 100, 200 mg	q12–24h
Other brand names: Kadian	10, 20, 30, 40, 50, 60, 70, 80, 100, 130, 150, 200 mg ER	
Morphine Sulfate/ Naltrexone (Embeda)	20/.8, 30/1.2, 50/2, 60/2.4, 80/3.2, 100/4	q12–24h

(continued)

(*continued*)

Oxycodone	5, 10, 15, 20, 30 mg	High affinity for the κ-receptor
Oxycodone (Oxaydo)	5, 7.5 mg	Abuse deterrent features
Oxycodone/ acetaminophen (Roxicet)	5/325 mg 5/325/5 mL	q6h PRN
Oxycodone with APAP (Percocet, Endocet)	2.5/325 mg 5/325 mg 7.5/325 mg 10/325 mg	q4–6h PRN
Oxycodone/ Ibuprofen (Combunox)	5/400 mg	q6h PRN
Oxycodone/ Aspirin (Percodan)	4.8/325 mg	q6h PRN
Oxycodone/ acetaminophen (Xartemis XR)	7.5/325 mg	2 tabs q24h
Oxycodone (Xtampza) ER	9, 13.5, 15, 18, 27, 36 mg	q12h
Tramadol (Ultram)	50 mg	Weak μ-agonist; also good for neuropathic pain. High risk for serotonin syndrome when used with SSRIs.
Tramadol/APAP (Ultracet)	37.5/325 mg	
Buprenorphine (Butrans Patch)	5 mcg/hr 10 mcg/hr 15 mcg/hr 20 mcg/hr	Partial μ-receptor agonist and κ-antagonist
Buprenorphine (Belbuca)	75, 150, 300, 450, 600, 750, 900 mcg buccal strip	Partial μ-receptor agonist and κ-antagonist

(*continued*)

(*continued*)

OPIOID	DOSAGES	CONSIDERATIONS
Oxymorphone (Opana)	5, 10 mg	3x as potent as morphine q4–6h PRN
Oxymorphone (Opana) ER	5, 7.5, 10, 15, 20, 30, 40 mg	q12h
Oxycodone (Oxycontin)	10, 15, 20, 30, 40, 60, 80 mg	q12h
Tapentadol (Nucynta)	50, 75, 100 mg	q6h
Acetaminophen/ Caffeine/ Dihydrocodeine (Trezix)	320/30/16	q4–6h

APAP, acetaminophen; ER, extended-release; NMDA, N-methyl-D-aspartate; SSRI, selective serotonin reuptake inhibitor.

ANTISPASMODICS

ANTISPASMODIC	DOSAGES	CONSIDERATIONS
Tizanidine (Zanaflex)	2, 4, 6 mg 2–8 mg TID	May lower blood pressure. Good for spasticity secondary to a neurological injury. Suggested in women with chronic tension-type headache.
Baclofen	5–20 mg BID–QID	Titration (increasing or decreasing) of dosage should be done slowly. Baclofen withdrawal leads to pruritus, seizures, and irritability ("itchy, bitchy, twitchy").

(*continued*)

(*continued*)

Cyclobenzaprine (Flexeril)	10 mg TID	Most common side effect is drowsiness.
Dantrolene (Dantrium)	25, 50, 100 mg TID	Causes hepatotoxicity and requires frequent liver function tests
Methocarbamol (Robaxin)	500, 750 mg BID–TID	
Metaxalone (Skelaxin)	800 mg BID–TID	
Orphenadrine (Norflex)	100 mg BID	
Carisoprodol (Soma)	250–350 mg TID	High abuse potential

TRICYCLIC ANTIDEPRESSANTS

TCA	DOSAGES	CONSIDERATIONS
Amitriptyline (Elavil)	10–200 mg/d	Avoid in patients with cardiac arrhythmias and in the elderly.
Desipramine (Norpramin)	10–200 mg/d	
Doxepin HCL	10, 25, 50, 100 mg	
Imipramine (Tofranil)	10, 25, 50 mg	
Nortriptyline HCL (Pamelor)	10–200 mg/d	Better side-effect profile compared to amitriptyline

TCA, tricyclic antidepressants.

SELECTIVE SEROTONIN REUPTAKE INHIBITORS

SSRI	DOSAGES	CONSIDERATIONS
Citalopram (Celexa)	10, 20, 40 mg tabs	May not be useful for neuropathic agents compared to other antidepressants such as TCAs. SSRIs have been shown to provide analgesia in patients who also have symptoms consistent with depression.
Fluoxetine (Prozac)	10, 20, 30, 40 mg tabs	
Paroxetine (Paxil)	10, 20, 30, 40 mg tabs 12.5, 25, 37.5 mg tabs	
Sertraline (Zoloft)	25, 50, 100 mg tabs.	

SSRI, selective serotonin reuptake inhibitor; TCA, tricyclic antidepressants.

SEROTONIN–NOREPINEPHRINE REUPTAKE INHIBITOR

SNRI	DOSAGES	CONSIDERATIONS
Duloxetine (Cymbalta)	20, 30, 60 mg	QD or BID Maximum 120 mg/d
Milnacipran (Savella)	12.5, 25, 50, 100 mg	BID Maximum 200 mg/d

SNRI, serotonin–norepinephrine reuptake inhibitor.

OTHER ANTIDEPRESSANTS COMMONLY USED

ANTIDEPRESSANTS	DOSAGES	CONSIDERATIONS
Mirtazapine (Remeron)	30, 45 mg tabs	Helps with sleep disturbances and anxiety disorders
Nefazodone (Serzone)	100, 200 mg tabs	
Trazodone (Desyrel)	50, 100, 150 mg tabs	Helps with insomnia and depression
Venlafaxine (Effexor)	25, 37.5, 50, 75, 100 mg tabs	SNRI; may use in patients who are unable to tolerate TCAs; increases suicidality risk; increases blood pressure; used in patients diagnosed with CRPS.

CRPS, complex regional pain syndrome; SNRI, serotonin–norepinephrine reuptake inhibitor; TCA, tricyclic antidepressants.

ANTICONVULSANTS

ANTIEPILEPTICS	DOSAGES	CONSIDERATIONS
Gabapentin (Neurontin)	100, 300, 400, 600, 800 mg tabs Maximum 3,600 mg/d	Greatest side effect: somnolence. Requires renal dosing. Does not worsen renal function.
Pregabalin (Lyrica)	25, 50, 75, 100, 150, 300 mg tabs	Similar to gabapentin; more expensive
Carbamazepine (Tegretol)	200–600 mg tabs; Maximum 1,600 mg/d	Drug of choice for trigeminal neuralgia

(*continued*)

(continued)

ANTIEPILEPTICS	DOSAGES	CONSIDERATIONS
Phenytoin (Dilantin)	100, 200, 300 ER tabs	Requires monitoring of LFTs, CBC, and dilantin level
Valproic acid	250 mg tabs	Requires monitoring of CBC, LFTs, and dilantin level; causes nausea and sedation
Lamotrigine (Lamictal)	25, 50, 100, 200, 250 mg tabs	Limited use in neuropathic pain

CBC, complete blood count; LFT, liver function tests.

INTERVENTIONAL PHARMACOLOGY

Nerve blocks are performed for diagnostic and therapeutic purposes. When pain appears to cover multiple dermatomal levels, a selective nerve block may be performed to diagnose which dermatome or nerve is involved as the pain generator.

Rarely, a temporary nerve block may result in prolonged pain reduction. In cases of mechanical low back pain, a nerve block may disrupt the pain cycle and allow for rehabilitation and physical therapy to improve patient function.

Local Anesthetics

Adverse reactions include the following:

- Numbness of tongue or foreign taste
- Lightheadedness
- Auditory disturbances
- Muscle twitch
- Loss of consciousness
- Convulsions
- Coma
- Respiratory arrest
- Cardiovascular depression

LOCAL ANESTHETIC	CONCENTRATION	ONSET/DURATION
Lidocaine	.5%, 1%, 1.5%, 2%	Fast (30–60 min)
Bupivacaine	.25%, .5%, .75%	Slow (120–240 min)

CORTICOSTEROIDS

A variety of steroids are used to treat spinal pain and other types of painful conditions. Steroids inhibit the synthesis or release of proinflammatory substances causing reduction of inflammation.

The most common indication for corticosteroids in interventional pain management are in peripheral joints, extra-articular tissue such as bursa, and neuraxial structures and spaces such as facet joints and epidural space.

Radicular pain is more likely to respond to epidural steroid injections compared to mechanical low back pain.

Corticosteroids are associated with several common adverse reactions including hypertension, hyperglycemia, fluid retention, facial flushing, generalized erythema, depression, congestive heart failure, menstrual irregularities, gastritis, peptic ulcer disease, neural toxicity, hypothalamic–pituitary–adrenal axis suppression, Cushing's syndrome, bone demineralization, steroid myopathy, and allergic reactions.

COMMONLY USED AGENTS	HALF-LIFE	ANTI-INFLAMMATORY POTENCY	PARTICLE SIZE	NOTES
Hydrocortisone	8–12 hr	1		
Methylprednisolone	12–36 hr	5	<7.6 μ	Dense
Triamcinolone	12–36 hr	5	0.5–100 μ	Dense
Dexamethasone	36–72 hr	25		No platelet aggregation
Betamethasone	36–72 hr	25	Varied	

CONTRAINDICATIONS FOR CORTICOSTEROIDS IN INTERVENTIONAL PAIN MANAGEMENT

RELATIVE CONTRAINDICATIONS	ABSOLUTE CONTRAINDICATIONS
Joint instability	Bacteremia/Sepsis
Predisposition to bleeding	INR >1.4
Hemarthrosis	Septic joint
Uncontrolled diabetes	Osteomyelitis
Uncontrolled hypertension	Bacterial endocarditis
Fever	Blood thinners
Skin infection at the site of injection	

INR, international normalized ratio.

AMERICAN SOCIETY OF REGIONAL ANESTHESIA PREPROCEDURAL MANAGEMENT OF ANTICOAGULANTS AND ANTIPLATELETS

DRUGS	WHEN TO STOP	WHEN TO RESTART
ASA and NSAIDs		
ASA and ASA combinations	6 d	24 hr
Diclofenac	1 d	24 hr
Ketorolac	1 d	24 hr
Ibuprofen	1 d	24 hr
Indomethacin	2 d	24 hr
Etodolac	2 d	24 hr
Naproxen	4 d	24 hr

(continued)

(*continued*)

Meloxicam	4 d	24 hr
Nabumetone	6 d	24 hr
Oxaprozin	10 d	24 hr
Piroxicam	10 d	24 hr
Phosphodiesterase Inhibitors		
Cilostazol	2 d	24 hr
Dipyridamole	2 d	24 hr
Anticoagulants		
Warfarin	5 d, normal INR	24 hr
Acenocoumarol	3 d, normal INR	24 hr
IV heparin	4 hr	2 hr (24 hr if patient is high risk for postinjection bleed)
Subcutaneous heparin (BID and TID)	8–10 hr	2 hr (24 hr if patient is high risk for postinjection bleed)
LMWH: prophylactic	12 hr	4–24 hr (depending on high risk for postinjection bleed)
LMWH: therapeutic	24 hr	4–24 hr (depending on high risk for postinjection bleed)
Fibrinolytic Agents		
Fondaparinux	4 d	24 hr

(*continued*)

(*continued*)

DRUGS	WHEN TO STOP	WHEN TO RESTART
P2Y12 Inhibitors		
Clopidogrel	7 d	12–24 hr
Prasugrel	7–10 d	12–24 hr
Ticagrelor	5 d	12–24 hr
New Anticoagulants		
Dabigatran	4–5 d 6 d (impaired renal function)	24 hr
Rivaroxaban	3 d	23 hr
Apixaban	3–5 d	24 hr
Glycoprotein IIb/IIIa Inhibitors		
Abciximab	2–5 d	8–12 hr
Eptifibatide	8–24 hr	8–12 hr
Tirofiban	8–24 hr	8–12 hr

ASA, acetylsalicylic acid; ASRA, American Society of Regional Anesthesia; LMWH, low-molecular-weight heparin.

SCHEDULE MEDICATIONS

SCHEDULE I	SCHEDULE II	SCHEDULE III	SCHEDULE IV	SCHEDULE V
Illegal/restricted to research drugs	Requires Rx	Requires Rx	Requires prescription	Requires Rx or may be OTC
High abuse potential	High abuse potential	Moderate abuse potential	minimal—moderate abuse potential	Limited abuse potential
	No refills or verbal orders allowed	Five refills in 6 mo	Five refills in 6 mo	Maximum five refills/6 mo
		Verbal orders allowed	Verbal orders allowed	Verbal orders allowed
Hallucinogens	Amphetamines	Anabolic steroids	Benzodiazepines	Pregabalin
Heroin	Opioids (single)	Dronabinol	Sedatives/hypnotics	opioid-derivative antidiarrheals and antitussives.
	Barbiturates	Ketamine	Appetite suppressants	
		Opioids (some combinations)		

OTC, over-the-counter.

Cervical Spine

Cervical Spondylosis

DEFINITION: Cervical spondylosis is defined as osteoarthritis of the cervical spine, which may include the degeneration of either the disk or facet joints. Usually, this spontaneous degeneration may not lead to symptoms. It can lead to symptoms referable to the neck, leading to loss of joint motion, pain with range of motion, or joint incompetency. It can also lead to neurologic complications of advanced joint degeneration. The condition may also progress to causing increased pressure on the spinal cord (leading to cervical spondylotic myelopathy) and/or cervical spinal nerve roots (cervical spondylotic radiculopathy).

EPIDEMIOLOGY: Cervical spondylosis prevalence varies with age. MRI studies have revealed that nearly 100% of adults who are aged older than 40 years have degeneration of at least one cervical level out of which only a small subdivision of patients present with spontaneous degenerative disease.

RISK FACTORS: The causes of cervical spondylosis are due to spontaneous degenerative joint process, and likely related to "wear and tear." The cervical disk joint may become dehydrated causing disk space narrowing. Once a certain degree of narrowing occurs, the annulus of the disk can develop osteophytes at the margin. The facet joints are synovial joints and are relatively immobile joints. Their function is primarily to prevent excessive rotation, flexion, and extension. The degeneration of the facet is accelerated as the disc space narrows due to more stress on the facet joints.

COMPLICATIONS: Advanced disease and complications of cervical spondylosis can lead to cervical spondylotic radiculopathy or cervical spondylotic myelopathy.

When the cervical discs degenerate, raised margins approximate with the body of the superior vertebral body. The end result is the degenerative joint change called the joint of Luschka, which is also known as uncovertebral joint.

ASSESSMENT

- Axial neck pain includes elements of direct pain (particularly in the posterior aspects of the neck). Axial neck pain can also exist in any axial muscle, including trapezius, interscapular muscles, or cervical paraspinals, leading to recurrent muscle spasms.

- Patients may also complain of occipital headache as referred pain from cervical spondylosis.

- Spontaneous onset of neck pain is more likely to be associated with cervical spondylosis, especially if the patient suffers multiple episodes over time. If the neck pain is acute and associated with a specific event, cervical myofascial strain and/or trauma should be considered.

- Patients may also complain of weakness, numbness, and pain radiating down an arm, which may be signs and symptoms of cervical spondylotic radiculopathy or cervical spondylotic myelopathy.

- Neck pain following infection or a history of malignancy may suggest more serious conditions.

DIAGNOSTIC TESTS

- Cervical x-ray may be ordered, which may reveal degenerative joint disease or degenerative disc disease.

- Cervical MRI may be ordered, which may reveal destruction of bone, spinal cord, or nerve root compression. MRI is also sensitive for an intradural or epidural process. A CT scan/myelogram may be performed if MRI is contraindicated.

- Electrodiagnostic studies may also be ordered which may reveal a denervation process. Electrodiagnostic studies will also be helpful for localizing the nerve root and ruling out a peripheral nerve entrapment.

TREATMENT

- Treatment of acute neck pain that has been going on for less than 6 weeks includes physical therapy.

- Taking supine breaks may be helpful.

- Depending on severity of the neck pain, use of acetaminophen/ nonsteroidal anti-inflammatory drugs (NSAIDs) may be beneficial.

- If the patient endorses muscle spasms with pain, use of muscle relaxants and modalities such as heat, transcutaneous electrical nerve stimulation (TENS) units, and massage may be helpful.

- Excessive prolonged cervical extension should be avoided.
- Triggering activities should be avoided.
- Diagnostic and/or therapeutic medial branch blocks may be performed to confirm the diagnosis. A radiofrequency ablation of the cervical medial branches may be performed after one or two successful diagnostic medial branch blocks.

Cervical Radiculopathy

DEFINITION: Cervical radiculopathy is defined as dysfunction of a spinal nerve root emerging from the level of the cervical spine. It is commonly associated with a disc herniation. It usually presents with pain, numbness, and/or weakness in a specific radicular pattern. It has a variable presence of weakness, changes in the reflexes, and development of paresthesias leading to interferences of activities of daily living.

ETIOLOGY: Cervical radiculopathy is caused by nerve dysfunction due to compression such as inflammation, nerve tumors, herniated discs, neuroforaminal narrowing, trauma, and external tumors.

RISK FACTORS: Risk factors include individuals who perform manual labor that require lifting, motor vehicle accidents (whiplash injury), predisposition to degenerative disc disease, and smoking.

COMPLICATIONS: Secondary complications include loss of cervical range of motion, chronic headaches or neck pain, loss of cervical lordosis, and worsening of degenerative disc disease.

ASSESSMENT

- Important information during history requires establishment of the pain characteristics, the distribution of pain, intensity, factors aggravating and alleviating pain, causes of possible injury, and other joint or spine disease.
- Functional assessment evaluates how the pain or weakness affects the patient's ability to manage activities of daily living including personal care, lifting, ability to work, concentrate, sleep, and management of pain.
- Physical examination:
  1. Inspection: Check alignment, prior surgery scars, muscle atrophy, or skin defects.
  2. Palpation: Assess for local tenderness of the spinous processes, cervical paraspinals atrophy, and asymmetry.

3. Range of motion: Document range of motion in forward flexion, hyperextension, rotation bilaterally, and lateral bending bilaterally.

4. Special tests and provocative maneuvers:

   a. Spurling's test is a foraminal compression test performed by extending and rotating the head toward the side being tested and then axial loading by applying a downward pressure on the head. The test is considered positive if the pain radiates into the arm ipsilaterally.

   b. Shoulder abduction relief sign (Bakody) is active abduction of the symptomatic upper extremity, placing the patient's ipsilateral hand on head. Posttest is relief or reduction of ipsilateral cervical radicular symptoms.

   c. Lhermitte's sign is a cervical spinal cord compression test performed by cervical flexion or extension causing a shock-like sensation in the spinal axis and the arms.

ROOT	MUSCLE(S)	PRIMARY MOTION	SENSORY LANDMARKS	REFLEX
C5	Deltoid bicep	Shoulder abduction Elbow flexion	Lateral arm	Bicep
C6	Brachioradialis Extensor carpi radialis longus	Elbow flexion Wrist extension	Radial (lateral) forearm Thumb	Brachi-oradialis
C7	Triceps Flexor carpi radialis	Elbow extension Wrist flexion	Digits 2–4	Tricep
C8	Flexor digitorum superficialis	Finger flexion	Digit 5	
T1	Dorsal interossei of hand	Finger abduction	Medial elbow	

  d. Hoffman's test is a test performed by holding the middle phalanx of the long finger and then flicking the distal phalanx into an extended position. If the thumb interphalangeal joint involuntarily contracts, the test is considered positive. It is indicative of cervical myelopathy due to possible damage to the anterior horn cell.

DIAGNOSTIC STUDIES

- Imaging:
  1. X-rays offer low sensitivity due to inability to visualize soft structures such as detection of nerve root compression or disc herniation. X-ray may show disc space narrowing, subchondral sclerosis, and formation of osteophytes. An open mouth x-ray may be required to rule out atlantoaxial instability and to visualize upper cervical levels.
  2. MRI is the imaging of choice and is indicated in persistent signs and symptoms for greater than 3 to 4 weeks of conservative management or worsening of symptoms such as progressive neurological function loss.
  3. MRI with and without gadolinium is indicated in cases of malignancy, infection, and postsurgery. Gadolinium with "light up" differently in cases where tumor, infection, abscess, or scar tissue is present.
  4. CT scan or CT myelogram may be performed if MRI is contraindicated.
- Nerve conduction studies (NCS) and electromyography (EMG) may be performed to distinguish which nerve root(s) may be affected. NCS may show decreased amplitude or normal responses. EMG is more diagnostic, and shows spontaneous potential, abnormal insertional activity such as positive sharp waves and fibrillation potentials. EMG testing of the cervical paraspinal muscles is very sensitive for cervical radiculopathy and/or myelopathy. EMG is usually negative for pathology in the first 3 to 4 weeks after symptom onset, and should not be ordered unless symptom onset is greater than 4 weeks.
- Electrodiagnostic protocol for cervical radiculopathy:
  1. NCS: Minimum of one motor NCS and one sensory NCS in the symptomatic extremity to determine if other concomitant

nerve disorder is present. Sensory nerve action potentials (SNAPs) should be normal in radiculopathy.

a. Compound muscle action potential (CMAP)/SNAP of median or ulnar nerve of the symptomatic side

OR

b. CMAP/SNAP of bilateral upper extremities median and ulnar nerve, and a peripheral nerve of the lower extremity of polyneuropathy is suspected.

c. Flexor carpi radialis (FCR) H-reflex if C7 radiculopathy is suspected.

d. F-wave—ulnar and median studies if C8 or T1 radiculopathy suspected.

2. EMG:

a. Test five or more muscles in the symptomatic side covering all myotomes ± paraspinals of the suspected spinal level.

b. Test one to two muscles innervated by the suspected root level and different peripheral nerves.

c. If a muscle is abnormal, consider testing the contralateral muscle.

3. Recommended EMG muscles:

MUSCLE	NERVE	C5	C6	C7	C8	T1
Rhomboids	Dorsal scapular	*				
Deltoids	Axillary	*	*			
Bicep	Musculocutaneous	*	*			
Brachioradialis	Radial	*	*			
FCR	Median		*	*		
Pronator teres	Median		*	*		
APB	Median				*	*
Tricep	Radial		*	*	*	
EIP	PIN			*	*	
FCU	Ulnar			*	*	*

(continued)

(*continued*)

MUSCLE	NERVE	C5	C6	C7	C8	T1
FDI	Ulnar			*	*	*
Pronator quadratus	AIN				*	*

AIN = anterior interosseous nerve; APB = abductor pollicis brevis; EIP = extensor indicis proprius; FCR = flexor carpi radialis; FCU = flexor carpi ulnaris; FDI = first dorsal interosseous; PIN = posterior interosseous nerve.

TREATMENT

- Mild cases may be treated with NSAIDs, Tylenol, and topical medications.
- Medrol dose pack may be required for acute phases.
- Muscle relaxants and opiates may be used in refractory cases.
- Selective nerve root blocks, paravertebral blocks, epidural steroid injections may be used during acute or subacute cervical radiculopathy.
- Chronic pain management includes:
  1. NSAIDs
  2. Gabapentin/pregabalin
  3. Tricyclic antidepressants (TCA)
  4. Anxiolytics
  5. Compound creams
- Use of muscle relaxants should be used in patients with spasms or spasticity.
- Use of opioid analgesics should be limited in chronic pain management.
- If chronic pain is significantly interfering with sleep and activities of daily living, an interdisciplinary approach with should implemented.

REHABILITATION REGIMEN

- Goal: Pain reduction, functional improvement, increase pain-free range of motion
- Modalities: Ice, heat, TENS units, electrical stimulation
- Progressive stretching in full range of motion (ROM) of cervical spine

- Strengthening of cervical stabilizers, shoulder girdle, and back muscles

- Development of a home exercise regimen

- Activity modification/ergonomics:
  1. Reduction of cervical strain by not flexing the neck while using a phone, tablet, or book
  2. No reading or watching TV while in bed to limit flexion
  3. One pillow use at night
  4. Limited use of traditional bifocals while using computer because it may cause hyperextension of the neck

INTERDISCIPLINARY COORDINATION OF CARE

- Surgery (orthopedic or neurosurgery), psychology, psychiatry, support groups, physical, and occupational therapies may all play a role.

- Infectious disease, oncology, urology, and plastic surgery may also play a role depending on the etiology and severity of the condition.

Cervical Spondylotic Myelopathy

DEFINITION: Traumatic compression of the cervical spinal cord or spinal cord ischemia due to arterial compression, and/or other consequences of cervical spondylosis. It may result from degenerative changes of the cervical spine, including facet joint degenerative changes. It may also occur from a congenitally narrow spinal canal that may cause predisposed changes to the spine.

Most common cause of spinal cord dysfunction in patients over the age of 55. It is commonly seen in C5 to C7 segments are more frequently involved.

STATIC FACTORS CONTRIBUTING TO MYELOPATHY	DYNAMIC FACTORS CONTRIBUTING TO MYELOPATHY
• Reactive hypertrophy, osteophyte formation at endplates • Hypertrophy of facet joints and ligamentum flavum • Decreased intervertebral height	• Ligamentum flavum buckling into the spinal column with hyperextension • Reactive hypermobility of adjacent spinal segments causing cord impingement

Onset is usually gradual unless secondary to an injury (i.e., whip-lash, hyperextension of C-spine).

Neurological symptoms related to motor weakness occurs faster and less likely to improve compared to sensory abnormalities. Imbalance may occur if the myelopathy goes unaddressed. Imbalance is slow to recover after intervention.

ASSESSMENT

- In addition to obtaining detail about pain and progression of the symptoms, it is important to evaluate changes in function, gait, balance, and loss of fine motor skills to evaluate where in the disease progression gradient the patient is currently. Assessment of injury and/or collision should be evaluated as well.

- Muscle atrophy and/or fasciculations may be seen. Upper motor signs (Hoffman, Babinski, hyperreflexia, and/or clonus) are indicative of cord compression.

- Central cord syndrome (spinal cord injury) may occur in patients with a hyperextension injury where patients typically have greater weakness in upper extremities compared to lower extremity weakness.

- Physical examination:

  1. Gait, fall risks, and balance assessments should be done in addition to what was discussed in the cervical stenosis section.

  2. Gait and balance

     a. Toe-to-heel walk will be difficult for the patient to perform.

     b. Romberg's test should be performed with the patient standing with arms held forward and eyes closed. The test is positive, suggesting that sensory ataxia is present, and that there is loss of proprioception.

  3. Special tests

     a. Spurling's test is a foraminal compression test performed by extended and rotated the head toward the side being tested and then axial loading by applying a downward pressure on the head. The test is considered positive if the pain radiates into the arm ipsilaterally.

     b. Lhermitte's sign is a cervical spinal cord compression test performed by cervical flexion or extension causing a shock-like sensation in the spinal axis and the arms.

     c. Hoffman's test is a test performed by holding the middle phalanx of the long finger and then flicking the distal phalanx into an extended position. If the thumb inter-phalangeal joint involuntarily contracts, the test is considered positive. It is indicative of cervical myelopathy due to possible damage to the anterior horn cell.

- Classification of myelopathy:

  1. Nurick classification

Grade 0	Signs or symptoms of root involvement without spinal cord disease
Grade 1	Signs of spinal cord disease without difficulty in walking
Grade 2	Difficulty in walking without effect on employment
Grade 3	Difficulty in walking with effect on full-time employment
Grade 4	Can walk only with an aid or walker
Grade 5	Chair bound or bedridden

  2. Ranawat classification

Class I	No neural deficits
Class II	Subjective weakness, dysesthesia, and hyperreflexia
Class IIIA	Objective weakness and long tract signs; patient is ambulatory
Class IIIB	Objective weakness and long tract signs; patient is no longer ambulatory

IMAGING

- Cervical anteroposterior (AP) x-rays may reveal degenerative changes of the Luschka's joints (uncovertebral or neurocentral joints) and facet joints, formation of osteophytes, disc space narrowing, and decreased sagittal diameter. If the diameter is less than 13 mm, cord compression may occur.

- A lateral radiograph may be performed to assess the diameter of the spinal canal, and obtain a Torg–Pavlov ratio. The Torg–Pavlov ratio is defined as the ratio between the sagittal diameter of the cervical canal to the width of the cervical vertebral body. Less than .80 seen on the lateral view indicates presence of cervical stenosis.

- Obtain lateral flexion and extension x-rays to assess range of motion and instability and to assess for angular or translational instability.

- An oblique x-ray may also assess for foraminal stenosis which may be due to degenerative changes of the Luschka's joints.

Red flags in spinal pain indicate that there may be a serious or life-threatening cause of back pain and will require further work up.

Yellow flags include poor sleep, avoidance of normal activity and extended rest, catastrophic thinking (thoughts of hurting self or others), there is no way the patient can control the pain, disaster will occur if the pain continues, expectation that pain will worsen with increased activity or work, increased stress and anxiety, compensation and work issues, poor job satisfaction, extended time off work, and poor relationship with supervisors.

INFECTION	MALIGNANCY (METASTASIS)	CAUDA EQUINA
• History of IV drug abuse • Recent spine surgery within the last 12 months • Fever and chills • Recent bacterial infection (wounds, lung, skin, UTI, pyelonephritis) • Immunocompromised	• Weight loss • Pain worse at night or at rest • Prior history of cancer	• Saddle anesthesia • Urine incontinence • Fecal incontinence • Decreased anal sphincter tone • Worsening of weakness and numbness • Progressive neurological deficits

IV, intravenous; UTI, urinary tract infection.

Cervical Spinal Stenosis

DEFINITION: Absolute stenosis defined as less than 10 mm; relative stenosis is defined as less than 13 mm.

- Congenital: Seen in younger and athletic patients.
    1. Associated with shorter pedicle and lateral laminae anomalies.
- Degenerative: Seen in middle-aged to older patients.
    1. Results from degenerative disk and facet disease associated with aging. Aging also leads to uncinate process hypertrophy, ligamentum flavum thickening, and the posterior longitudinal ligament may buckle.

Average AP diameter of the spinal canal measures approximately 17 mm to 18 mm in the mid-cervical segments. The space required by the spinal cord is approximately 9 mm to 10 mm.

Risk factors for development of cervical stenosis include sports participation, specifically soccer, football, rugby, other contact sports, and horseback riding. History of major whiplash trauma or dystonia may also lead to cervical stenosis.

The disease may progress from cervical stenosis to cervical myelopathy variably in all patients, and is difficult to predict. Many patients may experience axial neck pain periodically while others may experience symptoms of radiculitis and/or radiculopathy. Some patients may develop myelopathy with gait and balance impairment, bowel or bladder dysfunction, and/or loss of fine motor skills.

Ischemia or mechanical insults to the spinal cord from cervical stenosis may lead to neuronal damage.

ASSESSMENT

- In addition to obtaining details about pain and progression of the symptoms, it is important to evaluate changes in function, gait, balance, and loss of fine motor skills to evaluate where in the disease progression gradient the patient is currently. Assessment of injury and/or collision should be evaluated as well.

- Functional assessment evaluates how the pain or weakness affects the patient's ability to manage activities of daily living including personal care, lifting, ability to work, concentrate, sleep, and management of pain. The gait may be wide based. If myelopathy is present, other signs and symptoms include muscle wasting, loss of dexterity, numbness, and intrinsic muscle wasting. Bowel and bladder dysfunction is typically a late manifestation.

STUDIES

- Imaging: Cervical spine radiographs may be ordered in patients with suspected cervical stenosis. The Torg–Pavlov ratio is defined as the ratio between the sagittal diameter of the cervical canal to the width of the cervical vertebral body. Less than .80 seen on the lateral view indicates presence of cervical stenosis. Due to a relative high false positive rate, an MRI of the cervical spine should also be ordered.
- Electrodiagnostic tests may be useful in patients where the differential diagnosis includes a peripheral mononeuropathy or polyneuropathy or a motor neuron disease.
- Ergonomic evaluation of patient's workplace may also be necessary if symptoms are worse while at work. This will allow the patient to request an ergonomic workstation, improvement of postural alignment, and to decrease stress on the cervical spine.

MEDICATION MANAGEMENT

- Treatment is usually conservative for pain if no myelopathic symptoms present. NSAIDs and Tylenol may be used at regular intervals. A short course of opioids and/or muscle relaxants may be used in more severe cases.
- Steroid packs may be used in patients with functionally limiting pain with a 7- to 10-day steroid taper.
- Neuropathic pain medications may be used for patients with radicular pain. Gabapentin, pregabalin, TCAs are usually first-line agents.

REHABILITATION PROGRAM

- Goal: pain reduction, functional improvement, increase pain-free range of motion
- Modalities: ice, heat, TENS, massage, E-stim
- Avoidance of extreme cervical flexion and extension
- Stretching of the cervical spine, isometric exercises only during painful phase. Followed by strengthening, isotonic exercises once pain-free range of motion is achieved.
- Development of a home exercise program

Cervical Facet Mediated Pain

Cervical facet joint pain refers to pain originating from the facet joints (also known as zygapophyseal joints) in the cervical spine. It results from degeneration of the joint architecture, biomechanics, or function.

Facet syndrome results from abnormal loading and excessive stress on the facet joints secondary to trauma (whiplash injury), poor posture, disruption of the spine mechanics, fracture, inflammation/inflammatory disease, degenerative disc changes, degenerative facet arthropathy, and/or spondylolisthesis.

PATHOPHYSIOLOGY: The facet joints of the cervical spine are diarthrodial synovial joints. The joint capsules in the lower cervical spine are more mobile compared to other areas of the spine to allow a smooth gliding movement of the facet. The joints' alignment prevents excessive anterior translation and an important factor in weight bearing. The facet joints of the cervical spine are supplied by both the anterior and dorsal rami. The occipitoatlantal joint and the atlantoaxial joint are innervated by the ventral rami of the first and second spinal nerve. Two branches from the dorsal ramus of the third cervical spinal nerve innervate the C2–C3 facet joint. Facet joints from C3–C4 to C7–T1 are supplied by the dorsal rami medial branches that arise one level cephalad and caudad to the joint, leading to the joint being innervated by its medial branches above and below. The distance between the nerves and the bone is approximately 2 mm to 3 mm.

Facet arthropathy pain radiation (Figure 4.1 and Table 4.1):

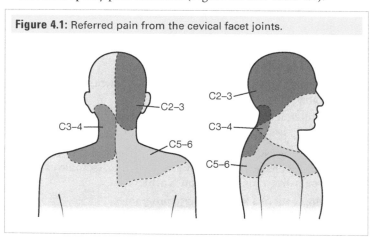

Figure 4.1: Referred pain from the cevical facet joints.

TABLE 4.1: INNERVATION OF CERVICOTHORACIC FACET JOINTS

FACET JOINT	INNERVATION
C2–C3	C2/C3 (third occipital nerve) and C3 medial branch
C3–C4	C3 and C4 medial branches
C4–C5	C4 and C5 medial branch
C5–C6	C5 and C6 medial branch
C6–C7	C6 and C7 medial branch
C7–T1	C7 and C8 medial branch
T1–T2	C8 and T1 medial branch

DISEASE STAGES

- Acute: occurs over 1 to 4 weeks, and is characterized by minor functional limitations, specifically abnormal motion causing pain. Other clinical features may include muscle spasm
- Subacute: occurs over 1 to 3 months, and is secondary to further degeneration and laxity of the facet joint resulting in prolonged periods of pain
- Chronic/stable: greater than 3 months, associated with osteophyte formation which is the body's effort to stabilize the motion at the affected joint

COMPLICATIONS: Facet hypertrophy may cause impingement of the spinal nerve leading to radiculitis and progress to radiculopathy. Facet arthropathy, specifically with involvement of the C1–C2 and C2–C3 joints may cause headaches.

ASSESSMENT

- Patients with cervical facet arthropathy will complain of neck pain, headaches, and limited range of motion. They will describe nonradicular pain which is dull and achy discomfort in the posterior neck which may radiate to shoulder or mid-back regions. Patients may have a previous history of a whiplash. Assessment of injury and/or collision should be inquired as well.
- Inspection may reveal increased or decreased lordosis, postural asymmetry. Physical examination may include tenderness to

palpation of the facet joints or paraspinal muscles. There may be pain with cervical extension and lateral rotation. Positive pain on extension or repetitive end-range extension is characteristic of facet mediated pain (facet-loading maneuvers).

COMMONLY PERFORMED PROCEDURES IN THE CERVICAL SPINE

Cervical Interlaminar Epidural Injection

INDICATIONS: Cervical stenosis, cervical radiculopathy, cervical disc herniation

CONTRAINDICATIONS

- Absolute contraindications:
  1. Patient refusal
  2. Local or systemic infection
  3. Spinal cord compression at the desired level of injection (spinal diameter <6 mm–7 mm with symptoms of cervical myelopathy)
  4. Inadequate treatment of bleeding disorders which predispose to hemorrhage
  5. Allergy to medications or contrast used
- Relative contraindications:
  1. Immunosuppressive state
  2. Pregnancy
  3. Inability to lie down (especially in conditions which may cause respiratory distress)
  4. Untreated hypertension
  5. Untreated diabetes
  6. Concurrent use of anticoagulation or antiplatelet agents, which may lead to bleeding and/or hematoma formation

FUNCTIONAL ANATOMY

- Cervical spine starts from the base of the skull and contains seven vertebrae, labeled C1–C7.
- The cervical nerves exit from the intervertebral neural foramen, and are labeled C1–C8.

EPIDURAL SPACE BOUNDARIES

Anteriorly	Posterior longitudinal ligament, vertebral discs, and bodies
Posteriorly	Ligamentum flavum, capsule of facet joints, and laminae
Laterally	Pedicles and intervertebral foramina
Superiorly	Fusion of the spinal and periosteal layers of dura mater at the foramen magnum
Inferiorly	Sacrococcygeal membranes

- Order of encountered structures while performing a cervical interlaminar epidural injection:
  1. Skin
  2. Subcutaneous tissue
  3. Ligamentum nuchae or supraspinous ligament
  4. Interspinous ligament
  5. Ligamentum flavum
  6. Epidural space

RECOMMENDED NEEDLE: 18- or 20-gauge needle, 2½ or 3½ inch Tuohy needle

INJECTATE: 2 mL to 3 mL normal saline, 12 mg betamethasone, 10 mg dexamethasone, or 40 mg triamcinolone

CONTRAST VOLUME: 2 mL to 4 mL

PATIENT POSITIONING

- Place the patient in a prone position on the C-arm table.
- A roll or pillows are placed under the patient's chest to induce a mild flexion of the cervical spine and to open the interlaminar space.

TECHNIQUE

- Rotate the C-arm so the spinous processes are aligned midline in AP, and tilt the C-arm caudally so the end plates are aligned to show a single solid line rather than two individual lines.

- Prep the skin using a chlorhexidine prep (preferably), povidone iodine, or isopropyl alcohol, which are all options for antiseptic agents for use in percutaneous spine procedures.

- Identify the appropriate interlaminar space with fluoroscopy using a radiopaque object such as a needle, using a metal marker to mark the space. Use a sterile marker if using a marker.

- Infiltrate the skin and subcutaneous tissues with 3 mL to 5 mL of 1% lidocaine using a 25- or 27-gauge needle. Inject into the deeper ligamentous structures for a better anesthetic effect.

- With the C-arm in the AP position, the Tuohy needle is introduced midline approach with the tip of the needle directed toward the midline between spinous process of the level desired or to the ipsilateral side of the patient's pain.

- Advance the needle slowly with frequent confirmations of not crossing midline using the C-arm.

- The needle is advanced until the interspinous ligament is "subjectively" encountered.

- The C-arm is then rotated into a lateral position to allow confirmation of the depth.

- Now, based on the practitioner's preference, a loss of resistance (using air or saline) technique can be utilized to identify entrance into the epidural space. The needle stylet is removed and a syringe with either saline or air is attached to the hub of the needle.

- The needle is stabilized by holding the wings and advanced slowly in the same trajectory and the "loss of resistance" is checked by gently tapping on the syringe plunger. Once the loss of resistance has occurred, the advancement of the needle should be stopped to prevent a "wet tap" or spinal cord injury. Needle advancement should be stopped if the patient develops severe pain or paresthesias. Make sure there is negative aspirate for air, cerebrospinal fluid (CSF), and blood.

  1. Caution: A small portion of the population **do not have ligamentum flavum** in the cervical spine, thus one may never feel that they are engaged in the ligament and a true (distinct) loss may not be present. This is why the level C7T1 is recommended.

- A negative aspiration check should be performed to ensure the needle is not placed into a blood vessel or for CSF. Connect the extension tubing to the needle and under live fluoroscopy, confirmation of epidural space entrance is verified by injection of

0.5 mL to 2 mL of nonionic contrast to verify spread into the epidural space by obtaining both lateral and AP views.

- Digital subtraction can also be utilized to ensure absence of vascular flow.
- After contrast confirmation of entry into the epidural space is done, the injectant mixture of corticosteroids and anesthetic is slowly injected.
- The stylet is then reinserted into the needle, and the needle is withdrawn slowly.
- Place a gauze on the needle entry point and apply pressure if there is bleeding. Place the sterile dressing or bandage of needle entry point.
- Observe the patient postprocedure to assure that there are no adverse reactions. Provide the patient with postprocedure care instructions.

COMPLICATIONS

- Mild complications include self-limited bleeding, which may induce postprocedure pain.
- Patient may also note myalgias or burning at the injection site several hours after the procedure due to the needle trauma.
- Postdural puncture ("wet tap") headache is an another potential complication where the patient complains of headache that gets better after lying down. A blood patch may be indicated if the headache does not improve.
- Postprocedure hyperglycemia may also occur secondary to corticosteroids. Patients who are diabetics should be aware of this to determine if their diet and/or insulin regimen needs to be adjusted after the procedure.
- More serious complications include:
  1. Epidural hematoma formation
  2. Arachnoiditis
  3. Intravascular injection → spinal cord ischemia
  4. Spinal cord injury
  5. Nerve root injury
  6. Pneumothorax
  7. Epidural abscess
  8. Osteomyelitis

Sample Procedure Note

PROCEDURE NOTE CERVICAL EPIDURAL STEROID

PREOPERATIVE DIAGNOSIS:	Cervical radiculitis cervical disc displacement cervicalgia
POSTOPERATIVE DIAGNOSIS:	Same
SURGEON:	_____
ASSISTANT:	_____
TITLE OF PROCEDURE:	_____ Cervical epidural steroid injection under fluoroscopic guidance (Video 4.1)

https://bcove.video/2IfO2RJ

Cervical Epidurogram Interpretation Under Fluoroscopy

ANESTHESIA:	Monitored anesthesia care
ESTIMATED BLOOD LOSS:	None
COMPLICATIONS:	None
DRAINS:	None
IV FLUID:	200 mL lactated ringer

Indications: _____-year-old _____ (male/female) complaining of cervical spine pain that radiates to the upper extremity. Our plan is to perform a cervical epidural steroid injection under fluoroscopic guidance today. The risks and benefits of _____ cervical epidural steroid injection were discussed in detail. The patient understands and accepts that the risks include, but are not limited to, increase in pain, nerve injury, infection, bleeding, hematoma, paralysis, spinal headache, stroke, discitis, and death. Alternatives to nerve blocks, or noninterventional therapy, were discussed and informed consent obtained.

DESCRIPTION OF PROCEDURE

Intravenous access was established. The patient was escorted to the fluoroscopy suite and placed in the prone position. Noninvasive monitoring was applied. Universal Site and Side Protocol was followed and documented. Safe Injection and

(continued)

(continued)

Infection Control Practices as recommended by the Center for Disease Control, including the use of a face mask, were strictly followed. The cervical area is widely prepped using isopropyl alcohol per protocol, and sterile drapes applied. Time-out was performed. Using fluoroscopic guidance, the cervical vertebral bodies were identified. Using a 25-gauge needle, a skin wheal was raised with 1% lidocaine. Under fluoroscopic guidance in the AP and lateral views, an 18-gauge modified winged Tuohy needle was placed at the _____ interspace. The Tuohy needle was advanced to the epidural space using intermittent loss of resistance technique with saline to identify the epidural space. Once the epidural space was identified AP and lateral projections of the fluoroscope confirmed adequate needle placement. At this point, 2 mL of Omnipaque-240 contrast was injected under live fluoroscopic guidance outlining a positive epidurogram. There was no evidence of intrathecal or intravascular spread. After negative aspiration for heme and CSF, 40 mg of Kenalog was injected with _____ mL of preservative-free sterile normal saline without complication. Once the procedure was completed all needles were withdrawn from the patient intact. A bandage was applied to the puncture site. The patient tolerated this procedure well, there were no complications noted. The patient was discharged home in hemodynamically and neurologically stable condition, with review of postprocedural instructions.

Plan: If the patient receives 50% or greater improvement of their pain we will repeat the procedure in 2 to 4 weeks' time. If today's injection does not alleviate the patient's pain by 50% we will perform a diagnostic cervical medial branch block under fluoroscopic guidance in 23 weeks.

Attending Physician

OPTIMAL IMAGES (Figures 4.2 and 4.3)

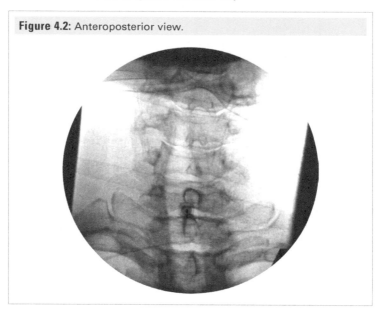

Figure 4.2: Anteroposterior view.

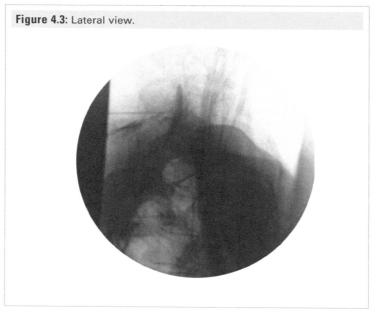

Figure 4.3: Lateral view.

CERVICAL MEDIAL BRANCH BLOCKS

FUNCTIONAL ANATOMY

- The cervical medial branch curves around articular process of the same vertebra and divides into ascending and descending branches. The branch is covered by tendons of the semispinalis muscles.

- The centroid of the articular process is higher.

- There are no cutaneous branches at the C4–C7 levels.

- Branches to the cervical facet joints are from the posterior portion of the medial branch. Therefore, creating a lesion anteriorly to the midportion of the articular process is important.

POSTERIOR APPROACH TECHNIQUE

- Place the patient in a prone position on the C-arm table for the posterior approach. A pillow may be placed under the patient's chest. The head is looking downward in a neutral position or to the opposite side of needle insertion.

- With the C-arm, obtain an AP view to identify the posterior aspect of the articular processes (articular pillars). Tilt the C-arm caudally. In this position, the beam runs parallel with the exiting nerve root. The goal of this set up is to line up the superior articular border with the inferior articular border.

- Clean the skin using a chlorhexidine prep or povidone iodine, both are equally effective antiseptic agents for use in percutaneous spine procedures.

- After identification of the levels to be blocked, a 22- or 25-gauge, 2- to 3-inch spinal needle can be inserted through the skin.

- Advance the needle with frequent fluoroscopy checks. Once the needle reaches the bone, it can be retracted slightly and the trajectory can be placed laterally to the deepest concave point, the location of the medial branches. The needle point should be at the lateral margin of the articular process.

- After a negative aspiration, inject local anesthetic. Contrast may also be used for further confirmation.

- Note: The C8 medial branch is blocked by placing the needle tip on the superior lateral border of the transverse process of T1.

- The patient should be instructed to assess his or her pain relief in 30 minutes to 1 hour increments immediately following the diagnostic blocks. The patient should also be instructed to not modify their activity postprocedure to ensure authentic results. A positive diagnostic block should demonstrate at least

50% reduction in pain. If successful, the procedure should be repeated at least one additional time to verify reproducibility before proceeding with a radiofrequency procedure.

- Complications:
  1. Transient neuritis and/or burning sensation in the treated spinal nerve
  2. Dural puncture
  3. Spinal cord trauma
  4. Spinal anesthesia
  5. Meningitis, neural trauma
  6. Pneumothorax
  7. Facet capsule rupture
  8. Hematoma formation

LATERAL APPROACH TECHNIQUE

- Place the patient in a supine or lateral decubitus (injection side up) for the lateral approach. Turn the head to the contralateral side to be injected, and the chin flexed. This allows an unobscured view of the cervical spine and opens up the ipsilateral facet joints.

- Tilt the C-arm caudal or cranial to align the facet joint of the appropriate level. The C-arm should be rotated oblique to align the lateral masses bilaterally. This view allows the facet joint to be in the same parallel orientation as the articular pillars waist, where the medial branch nerve lies.

- Using a curved 22- or 25-gauge spinal needle with a curved tip, aim for the lateral border of the articular pillars waist.

- Advance the needle by using a small lateral to medial approach, to make contact with the bone of the posterior pillar.

- Obtain a lateral view fluoroscopy image to confirm proper depth of the needle tip. The needle tip should be at the midpoint of the pillar.

- After a negative aspiration, inject local anesthetic. Contrast may also be used for further confirmation.

- The patient should be instructed to assess his or her pain relief in 30 minutes to 1 hour increments immediately following the diagnostic blocks. The patient should also be instructed to not modify their activity postprocedure to ensure authentic results. A positive diagnostic block should demonstrate at least 50% reduction in pain. If successful, the procedure should be repeated at least one additional time to verify reproducibility before proceeding with a radiofrequency procedure.

OPTIMAL IMAGES (Figures 4.4 and 4.5)

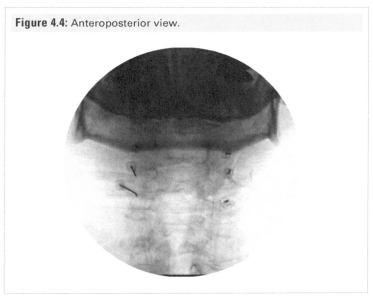

Figure 4.4: Anteroposterior view.

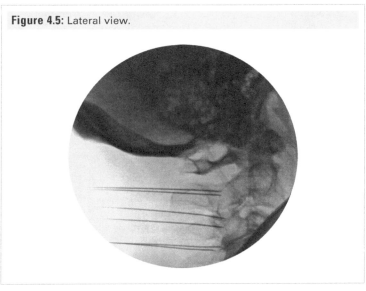

Figure 4.5: Lateral view.

Sample Procedure Note

PREOPERATIVE DIAGNOSIS: Cervical spondylosis

Cervical facet arthropathy

Cervicalgia

POSTOPERATIVE DIAGNOSIS: Same

SURGEON: _____

ASSISTANT: _____

TITLE OF PROCEDURE: Diagnostic _____ cervical medial branch block under fluoroscopic guidance **(Videos 4.2 and 4.3)**

https://bcove.video/2Ii0dcU

https://bcove.video/2wBUjSE

ANESTHESIA: Monitored anesthesia care

ESTIMATED BLOOD LOSS: None

COMPLICATIONS: None

DRAINS: None

IV Fluid: _____ mL lactated ringer

Indications: _____-year-old _____ (male/female) complaining of neck pain with reproducible facet tenderness to palpation. The pain does not radiate to the lower extremity. Our plan is to perform a diagnostic cervical medial branch block under fluoroscopic guidance today. The risks and benefits of _____ median branch nerve blocks were discussed in detail. The patient understands and accepts that the risks include, but are not limited to, increase in pain, nerve injury, infection, bleeding, hematoma, paralysis, spinal headache, stroke, discitis, and death. Alternatives to nerve blocks, or noninterventional therapy, were discussed and informed consent obtained.

DESCRIPTION OF PROCEDURE

Intravenous access was established. The patient was escorted to the fluoroscopy suite and placed in the prone position. Noninvasive monitoring was applied. Universal Site and Side Protocol was followed and documented. Safe Injection and

(continued)

(*continued*)

Infection Control Practices as recommended by the Center for Disease Control, including the use of a face mask, were strictly followed. The thoracic area is widely prepped using _____ per protocol, and sterile drapes applied. Time-out was performed. Using fluoroscopic guidance, the lateral borders and levels of _____ cervical bodies were identified and marked. Using a 25-gauge needle, a skin wheal was raised with 1% lidocaine. Under the fluoroscopic guidance, a 22-gauge 3.5-inch curved Quincke spinal needle was advanced to the midpoint of the centroids at the waist of the articular pillars of _____, where the median branch lies. AP and lateral projections of the fluoroscope confirmed adequate needle placement. There was no evidence of heme, CSF, or paresthesias noted at any time. At this point, 0.5 mL of Omnipaque contrast was injected under live fluoroscopic guidance outlining a well-defined neurogram through a T-Connector extension tubing. Then 0.5 mL of 0.75% bupivacaine (with/without Kenalog) was injected through the needle at each level to block the corresponding medial branch nerve utilizing a T-Connector extension tubing. At this point, all needles were withdrawn from the patient intact. A bandage was applied to the puncture site. The patient tolerated this sequence well, there were no complications noted. The patient was discharged in hemodynamically and neurologically stable condition with a pain diary and review of postprocedural instructions. We will follow up with the patient in our office for a possible radiofrequency ablation if they receive greater than 50% pain relief from today's procedure.

Attending Physician

Radiofrequency Ablation of the Cervical Medial Branches

INDICATIONS: After two successful medial branch block trials are done, an elective procedure with radiofrequency ablation of the medial branches may be offered to the patient for longer duration of desensitization of the facet joints. It is recommended that the diagnostic medial branch blocks should be performed twice using different local anesthetics for it to be truly diagnostic. The recommended volume is less than .30 mL for the cervical region at each locked.

CONTRAINDICATIONS

- Absolute contraindications:
  1. Patient refusal
  2. Local or systemic infection
  3. Spinal cord compression at the desired level of injection
  4. Inadequate treatment of bleeding disorders which predispose to hemorrhage
  5. Allergy to medications or contrast used
- Relative:
  1. Pacemaker, automated implantable cardio-defibrillators (AICD), spinal cord stimulator, or other devices which use radio frequency energy
  2. Poor or inadequate response prior to radiofrequency treatments
  3. Immunosuppressive state
  4. Pregnancy
  5. Inability to lie down (especially in conditions which may cause respiratory distress)
  6. Untreated hypertension
  7. Untreated diabetes
  8. Concurrent use of anticoagulation or antiplatelet agents which may lead to bleeding and/or hematoma formation

PATHOANATOMY: Each joint is innervated by a same level medial branch and one above level medial branch. Thus, to provide denervation of the entire joint, both of these medial branches need to be ablated.

TYPES

- Thermal: creates a sphere burn at approximately 80°C for approximately 60 to 90 seconds. This will lead to Wallerian degeneration of the medial branch approximately 2 to 3 weeks after the procedure.
- Pulsed: not always covered by insurance. Controversial for medial branch ablation. Creates a pinpoint pulsed burn causing stunning of the nerve. This is done between 40°C and 70°C for 240 pulses.

PROCEDURE: A lateral approach is recommended for pulsed radiofrequency lesions and a posterior approach is recommended for conventional radiofrequency lesions.

- Obtain an AP view of the appropriate level, and align the end plates by using caudal or cranial tilts.

- Infiltrate the skin and subcutaneous tissues with 3 mL to 5 mL of 1% lidocaine using a 25- or 27-gauge needle. Inject into the deeper ligamentous structures for a better anesthetic effect.

- Using a 20- or 22-gauge curved needle, either 5 cm or or 10 cm length, 5 mm active tip, advanced slowly with frequent fluoroscopy images, with the target point at the midpoint of the centroids at the waist of the articular pillar. Keep the curve of the needle facing medially toward the midline of the patient.

- Once the needle makes contact with the os, turn the needle curve away from the midline.

- Confirm depth with lateral view.

- Advance the needle to the trapezoid center of the vertebral body.

- Attach the radiofrequency needles with the RF generator.

- Testing prior to ablation:

  1. Sensory: Start 0 to 1 Hz. The patient may feel pressure or sensation below 1 Hz.

  2. Motor: Start 0 and advance to 2 Hz. You may observe the patient's multifidus contraction. If you observe muscle contraction or stimulation of the extremity, the needle may require repositioning.

- Inject local anesthetic once needle placement is confirmed by testing at each site.

- Start lesion 30 to 45 seconds after injecting the anesthetic.

- Next, combination of anesthetic and nonparticulate should be injected to prevent inflammation at the root.

COMPLICATIONS

- Bleeding
- Infection
- Percutaneous procedures
- Neuritis, dysesthesia, numbness
- If the third occipital nerve is involved, ataxia may also be observed

OPTIMAL IMAGES (Figures 4.6 and 4.7)

Figure 4.6: Anteroposterior view.

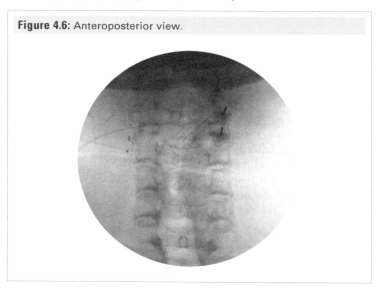

Figure 4.7: Lateral view.

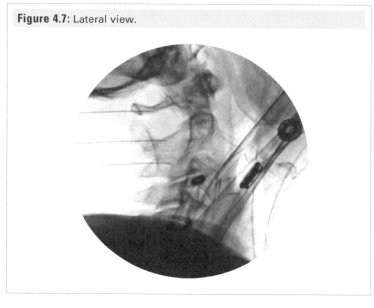

Sample Procedure Note

PREOPERATIVE DIAGNOSIS:	Cervical spondylosis
	Cervical facet
	arthropathy cervicalgia
POSTOPERATIVE DIAGNOSIS:	Same
SURGEON:	_____
ASSISTANT:	_____
TITLE OF PROCEDURE:	_____ Cervical
	radiofrequency thermal
	coagulation under
	fluoroscopic guidance
https://bcove.video/2IkaUvA	(**Video 4.4**)
ANESTHESIA:	Monitored anesthesia care
ESTIMATED BLOOD LOSS:	None
COMPLICATIONS:	None
DRAINS:	None
IV Fluid:	200 mL lactated ringer

Indications: _____-year-old _____ (male/female)
complaining of neck pain with reproducible facet tenderness
to palpation. The pain does not radiate to the upper extremity.
Our plan is to perform a cervical radiofrequency thermal
coagulation under fluoroscopic guidance today since the patient
reported greater than 50% pain relief with the diagnostic
cervical medial branch blocks that were previously completed.
The risks and benefits of _____ radiofrequency thermal
coagulation were discussed in detail. The patient understands
and accepts that the risks include, but are not limited to,
increase in pain, nerve injury, infection, bleeding, hematoma,
paralysis, spinal headache, stroke, discitis, and death.
Alternatives to nerve blocks, or noninterventional therapy, were
discussed and informed consent obtained.

DESCRIPTION OF PROCEDURE
Intravenous access was established. The patient was escorted
to the fluoroscopy suite and placed in the prone position.
Noninvasive monitoring was applied. Universal Site and Side
Protocol was followed and documented. Safe Injection and

(continued)

(*continued*)

Infection Control Practices as recommended by the Center for Disease Control, including the use of a face mask, were strictly followed. The thoracic area is widely prepped using _____ per protocol, and sterile drapes applied. Time-out was performed. Using fluoroscopic guidance, the lateral borders and levels of _____ cervical bodies were identified and marked. Using a 25-gauge needle, a skin wheal was raised with 1% lidocaine. Under the fluoroscopic guidance, a 22-gauge 10-cm length, 5-mm active tip, curved Neurotherm spinal needle was advanced to the midpoint of the centroids at the waist of the articular pillars of the _____, where the median branch lies. AP and lateral projections of the fluoroscope confirmed adequate needle placement. There was no evidence of heme, CSF, or paresthesias noted at any time. At this point, each needle was independently tested for sensory and motor stimulation. There was no radicular or nerve root stimulation noted at any time. There was concordant sensory overlap of the medial branch nerves. At this point 1 mL of 0.5% bupivacaine was injected through the needle at each level to block the corresponding medial branch nerve through a T-Connector extension tubing. Once 3 minutes had passed a thermal lesion was created at _____ levels at 80°C for 90 seconds. Once the lesion was complete 40 mg of Kenalog was injected in divided doses through a T-Connector extension tubing. At this point, all needles were withdrawn from the patient intact. A bandage was applied to the puncture site. The patient tolerated this sequence well, there were no complications noted. The patient was discharged in hemodynamically and neurologically stable condition, with review of postprocedural instructions. We will follow up with the patient in our office in 4 weeks.

_____

Attending Physician

Coding

PROCEDURES	CPT CODES
Cervical interlaminar epidural steroid injection	62321
Epidurogram	72275
Cervical transforaminal epidural steroid injection	64479
Additional levels	64480
Bilateral modifier	50
Epidurogram	72275
Cervical medial branch block or facet joint injection	64490
Second level	64491
Third level	64492
Bilateral modifier	50
RFA—First cervical level	64633
RFA additional levels	64634

Injectables	J-codes
Low osmolar contrast material (Omnipaque 300)	Q9967
Low osmolar contrast material (Omnipaque 240)	Q9966
Betamethasone (Celestone 3 mg)	J0702
Betamethasone (Celestone 4 mg)	J0704
Dexamethasone sodium phosphate 1 mg	J1100
Depo-Medrol (40 mg)	J1030
Depo-Medrol (80 mg)	J1040
Triamcinolone (per 10 mg)	J3301
Diphenhydramine (injection up to 50 mg)	J1200

(*continued*)

(*continued*)

Versed (per mg)	J2250
Fentanyl (0.1 mg)	J3010
Euflexxa (per dose)	J7323

RFA, radiofrequency ablation.

List of Videos

 Video 4.1 Cervical Epidural Steroid Injection

https://bcove.video/2IfO2RJ

Video 4.2 Cervical Medial Branch Block

https://bcove.video/2Ii0dcU

 Video 4.3 High Cervical Medial Branch Block

https://bcove.video/2wBUjSE

Video 4.4 High Cervical Radiofrequency Ablation

https://bcove.video/2IkaUvA

Thoracic Spine

THORACIC RADICULOPATHY/MYELOPATHY

DEFINITION: Thoracic radiculopathy is a disorder occurring in the neural elements between T1 and T12 level. It may occur from chemical irritation, metabolic abnormalities (i.e., diabetes, thyroid dysfunction), or mechanical compression. The majority of thoracic disc herniations occur between T8 and T12.

EPIDEMIOLOGY: It is uncommon and underdiagnosed because of a relative insufficient examination finding and due to its non-specific presentation. It is often overlooked during evaluation of spinal pain syndromes. Thoracic disc herniations are relatively common and often asymptomatic when compared to cervical or lumbar disc herniations. The thoracic region is relatively unyielding. Its primary function is to provide an erect posture and weight bear of the upper body during activities of daily living. Posture and weight-bearing functions of thoracic spine are assisted by the ribs, sternum, and ligamentous structures to provide additional support.

Due to its inflexible nature, thoracic intervertebral discs are more susceptible to injury when torsional and lateral forces are applied together.

The lower thoracic spine, from T8 to T12 is the most frequent site for thoracic radiculopathy. T11 to T12 interspace accounts for 25% to 50% of all thoracic herniations.

PATHOANATOMY

- The thoracic spinal canal has a smaller spinal canal clearance.

SYMPTOMS

- Most patients complain of "band-like" chest pain (Figure 5.1).
- If myelopathy is present, symptoms of upper motor neuron signs may be present. Evaluation of motor impairment, hyper-reflexia, spasticity, sensory impairment, and/or bowel or bladder dysfunction must be done.

Figure 5.1: Distribution of pain in thoracic radiculopathy.

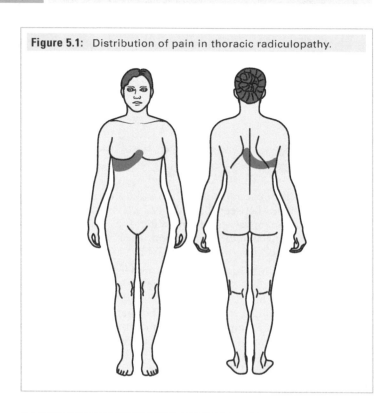

ROOT(S)	SYMPTOM
T2–T3	Axillary or midscapular pain
T7–T12	Abdominal pain
T11–12	Bowel or bladder dysfunction due to possible damage of the conus medullaris or cauda equina

ASSESSMENT

- Physical examination may show limitations of range of motion, particularly with trunk extension, flexion, and rotation secondary to pain and/or weakness. Range of motion should not be done repeatedly if a spinal fracture is suspected. Palpation to assess for tenderness over the ribs, intercostal spaces, thoracic transverse, and spinous processes are important in localizing the level involved in pain. If there is pain while palpating the vertebral bodies should warrant further workup for a possible vertebral fracture. Sensory examination may be also useful in localizing the level of injury.

ROOTS	SENSORY DISTRIBUTION
T2	Axillary, chest, upper medial aspect of arm
T4	Nipples
T10	Umbilicus
T12	Hip girdle

- Abnormality of the spine such as scoliosis should be noted when the patient flexes forward.
- Functional assessment from pain produced by thoracic radiculopathy should be assessed as well. Activities of daily living (ADLs) such as dressing, bathing, and putting on shoes may be difficult. Attempting work activities such as lifting and climbing may be restricted. Anorexia may also result from pain in the abdominal region.
- An ASIA score developed by the American Spinal Injury Association may be useful in neurologic assessment for patients who have suffered spinal cord injury from a traumatic cause. The score is able to assess the severity of the spinal cord injury.

DIAGNOSTIC STUDIES

- In patients with history of trauma or falls, plain x-rays should be ordered to rule out fractures or spinal instability.
- Due to the low incidence of thoracic radiculopathy/ myelopathy, there is a low threshold for obtaining imaging studies for patients who have had pain persisting greater than 3 to 4 weeks. MRI remains to be the gold standard to evaluate the thoracic spine and its soft neural structures. Gadolinium is useful to set forth a neoplasm, scar formation, or an infectious process. CT and/or CT myelogram are alternatives if MRI is contraindicated.

- Electrodiagnostic studies for thoracic radiculopathy are limited because of lack of easily accessible muscles in the thoracic myotomal distribution. The electromyographer may test paraspinals and intercostals. Abdominal muscles are not routinely tested. Multiple levels must be tested to localize the lesions.
- In cases where malignancy and metastasis is suspected, a PET scan may also be utilized to check for other foci of metastasis.

MEDICATION MANAGEMENT

- Mild cases may be treated with nonsteroidal anti-inflammatory drugs (NSAIDs), Tylenol, and topical medications.
- Medrol dose pack may be required for acute phases.
- Muscle relaxants and opiates may be used in refractory cases.
- Selective nerve root blocks, paravertebral blocks, intercostal nerve blocks, and epidural steroid injections may be used during acute or subacute thoracic radiculopathy.
- Chronic pain management includes the following
  1. NSAIDs
  2. Gabapentin/pregabalin.
  3. Tricyclic antidepressants (TCAs)
  4. Anxiolytics
  5. Compound creams
- Use of muscle relaxants should be used in patients with spasms or spasticity.
- Use of opioid analgesics should be limited in chronic pain management.
- If chronic pain is significantly interfering with sleep and activities of daily living, an interdisciplinary approach should be implemented.

REHABILITATION PROGRAM

- Goal: pain reduction, functional improvement, increase pain-free range of motion
- Modalities: ice, heat, transcutaneous electrical nerve stimulation (TENS) units, electrical stimulation, and ultrasound may also help reduce pain and improve modality.
- Physical therapy can progress with spine stabilization exercises, postural retraining, back and abdominal strengthening, and mechanical spinal traction.

- A thoracolumbar brace may be required to reduce spine movement. Should be used cautiously because it may cause muscle atrophy with prolonged use.
- Allodynia should be addressed with desensitization therapy, TENS.
- Development of a home exercise regimen
- Vocational therapy may help to maintain a productive life within the patient's limitations. Work sites can be evaluated, if indicated.

Red flags in spinal pain indicate that there may be a serious or life-threatening cause of back pain and will require further workup

INFECTION	MALIGNANCY (METASTASIS)	CAUDA EQUINA
<ul><li>History of IV drug abuse</li><li>Recent spine surgery within the last 12 months</li><li>Fever and chills</li><li>Recent bacterial infection (wounds, lung, skin, UTI, pyelonephritis)</li><li>Immuno-compromised</li></ul>	<ul><li>Weight loss</li><li>Pain worse at night or at rest</li><li>Prior history of cancer</li></ul>	<ul><li>Saddle anesthesia</li><li>Urine incontinence</li><li>Fecal incontinence</li><li>Decreased anal sphincter tone</li><li>Worsening of weakness and numbness</li><li>Progressive neurological deficits</li></ul>

IV, intravenous; UTI, urinary tract infection.

THORACIC COMPRESSION FRACTURE

Compression fractures of the spine usually result from conditions such as osteoporosis, trauma, excessive pressure, history of osteomyelitis, medications (specifically oral steroids, heparin, and/or anticonvulsants), or from a physical injury. If the bone in the spine collapses, it is defined as a vertebral compression fracture. Women are at an increased risk after menopause. Thin and frail individuals are also at an increased risk. Smoking can also increase the risk of this occurring.

Compression fractures typically occur in the thoracic spine. The most common location is T11 and T12, and the first lumbar vertebra, L1. Types of fractures described are wedge, biconcave, or crush fracture. Burst fractures result from high energy axial loading.

Compression fracture of the spine typically occurs from too much pressure on the vertebral body. It commonly occurs from bending forward and downward pressure on the spine.

Spinal compression fractures may shift the center of gravity forwardly, thus increasing the anterior load on the spine. The anterior load on the spine will increase the risk of a secondary compression fracture and/or fall.

Symptoms consist of severe pain in the back, legs, and/or arms. There may be also associated numbness and tingling if the fracture leads to injury to the nerves of the spine. If the bone collapse is more gradual, such as from bone thinning, the pain is typically on the milder side.

STAGING

- Acute: very painful
- Subacute: pain improves, mobility increases
- Chronic/stable: not much pain, prefracture function returns
- Preterminal: history of malignancy, respiratory dysfunction, gait abnormalities

Future fracture risk is elevated after the first compression fracture.

ASSESSMENT

- Important information during history requires establishment of the pain characteristics, previous fractures, history of aggressive physical activity, inappropriate training or equipment, and osteoporosis. The distribution of pain, intensity, factors aggravating and alleviating pain, radiation of the pain, bowel or bladder dysfunction, causes of possible injury, and other joint or spine disease. Pain with valsalva may also be indicative of a compression fracture. Observation of transfers may reveal guarding.

- Physical examination may show tenderness to palpation over an acute fracture.
- Discogenic provocative maneuvers are positive.

IMAGING

- Anteroposterior (AP) and lateral x-rays should be evaluated in all compression fractures. Wedge, crush, or biconcave fractures can be identified.
- MRI can be ordered in cases of high suspicion but negative x-rays. Gadolinium enhancement can be used to identify malignancies or infection.
- Bone scan may be an alternative in patients who cannot undergo MRI.
- CT scan is helpful to study bone detail, but will not measure acuity.
- Dual-energy x-ray absorptiometry (DEXA) scan may need to be done to evaluate for osteoporosis in other body parts.

REHABILITATION

- Assistive devices such as a single point cane or rolling walker may be used if mobility is limited.
- Braces
  1. Thoracic or lumbar compression fracture: TLSO or Jewett brace
  2. Physical therapy (PT) can help restore ADLs and start weight-bearing exercises with bracing.
  3. Pain medications may be used in acute stage.

CHEST WALL PAIN SYNDROME

Chest wall pain syndrome is defined as a painful state that presents as a direct or referred pain to the chest wall as a result of inflammation, stress, or injury to the body. More serious conditions such as acute coronary syndrome, pulmonary embolism, and pneumonia should be ruled out first.

Musculoskeletal conditions such as costochondritis, rib dysfunction, intercostal myalgia, sternoclavicular disease, intercostal neuralgia from shingles, seronegative spondyloarthropathies, myofascial pain, carcinoma, psoriatic arthritis, and/or postthoracotomy syndrome may lead to chest wall pain syndrome.

PATHOANATOMY

- The thorax is bordered by 12 ribs bilaterally, the sternum and the xiphoid anteriorly, 12 vertebrae posteriorly. These structures are interconnected with muscles and fascia. There are the anterior rami of the thoracic spinal nerves which form the intercostal nerves. The intercostal nerves course along the inferior border of the rib. Damage to the rib, the nerve, or muscle may cause impingement of the intercostal nerve. These nerve roots are also susceptible to dormant viruses and a potential site for shingles.

- Costochondritis is an inflammatory process of the cartilage that connects to the rib to the sternum. It presents as a pinpoint tenderness in the chest, localized over the costochondral joints along the sternum.

- Intercostal neuralgia is a painful disorder of the nerves that travel between the ribs and is secondary to damage or loss of function of one of the intercostal nerves. It results in burning, stabbing, and sharp discomfort in the dermatomal distribution. The most common cause for this is surgery.

- Shingles (postherpetic neuralgia) is reactivation of the varicella zoster virus resulting in burning/neuropathic pain with hyperesthesia followed by a vesicular rash. The rash may be limited to one or two dermatomes, and is unilateral.

- Assessment:
  1. A comprehensive pain history should be obtained after acute coronary syndrome, pulmonary embolism, pneumonia, and/or other life-threatening conditions have been ruled out.
  2. Assessment of the quality of pain, location, reproducibility, positional exacerbation, and previous events should be focused on.
  3. Physical examination:
     a. Auscultation of heart and lungs, palpation of the peripheral arteries
     b. Manual motor testing and inspection of the pectoral and scapular muscles
     c. Evaluation of range of movement (ROM) of shoulder and scapula should be performed.

    d. Palpation of the costochondral joints, ribs, and sternum

    e. Dermatomal sensory testing

    f. Evaluation of tender and trigger points of the levator scapulae, pectoralis major and minor, supraspinatus, infraspinatus, serratus anterior

4. Obtain an ECG, comprehensive metabolic panel (CMP), complete blood count (CBC), D-dimer, creatine kinase (CK)-MB, troponins, C-reactive protein (CRP), erythrocyte sedimentation rate (ESR), chest x-ray (CXR), abdominal x-ray (AXR), CT chest, should be performed to rule out acute and life-threatening etiologies. If in office setting, consider having the patient emergently transferred to the emergency room.

5. Rehabilitation and medication management:

    a. Costochondritis: physical therapy, modalities: ultrasound

    b. Rib fracture: intercostal nerve block, consider surgery consultation

    c. Postthoracotomy pain: paravertebral blocks, intercostal nerve blocks, trigger point injections, TCAs, gabapentin

    d. Intercostal neuralgia: TCAs, gabapentin, intercostal nerve block

    e. Postherpetic neuralgia: lidocaine patch, intercostal nerve block, gabapentin, pregabalin, TCAs, capsaicin, Qutenza patch

THORACIC INTERLAMINAR EPIDURAL STEROID INJECTION

INDICATIONS: Thoracic radiculopathy, thoracic herniated disc, stenosis of the thoracic spine

CONTRAINDICATIONS

- Absolute contraindications:

    1. Patient refusal

    2. Local or systemic infection

3. Spinal cord compression at the desired level of injection (spinal diameter less than 6–7 mm with symptoms of thoracic myelopathy)

4. Inadequate treatment of bleeding disorders which predispose to hemorrhage

5. Allergy to injectable medications

- Relative:

1. Immunosuppressive state

2. Pregnancy

3. Inability to lie prone (especially in conditions which may cause respiratory distress)

4. Untreated hypertension

5. Untreated diabetes

6. Concurrent use of anticoagulation or antiplatelet agents which may lead to bleeding and/or hematoma formation

TECHNIQUE

- Recommended needle: 18- or 20-gauge, 3½-inch Tuohy needle
- Injectate: 4 mL of normal saline and 10 mg of dexamethasone, 40 mg of triamcinolone, or 40 mg of Depo-methylprednisolone
- Contrast volume: 2 to 4 mL
- Patient positioning:

1. Place the patient in a prone position on the C-arm table.

2. Rotate the C-arm so the spinous processes are aligned midline in AP, and tilt the C-arm caudally so the end plates are aligned to show a single solid line rather than two individual lines. A slight oblique of the C-arm toward the symptomatic side may be done.

3. Prep the skin using a chlorhexidine prep (preferably), povidone iodine, and isopropyl alcohol are all options for antiseptic agents for use in percutaneous spine procedures.

4. Identify the appropriate interlaminar space with fluoroscopy using a radiopaque object such as a needle, metal marker to mark the space. Use a sterile marker if using a marker.

5. Infiltrate the skin and subcutaneous tissues with 2 mL to 4 mL of 1% lidocaine using a 25-gauge needle. Inject into the deeper ligamentous structures for a better anesthetic effect.

6. With the C-arm in the AP position, the Tuohy needle is introduced midline approach with the tip of the needle directed toward the midline between spinous process of the level desired or to the ipsilateral side of the patient's pain.

7. Advance the needle slowly with frequent confirmations of not crossing midline using the C-arm.

8. The needle is advanced until the interspinous ligament is "subjectively" encountered.

9. The C-arm is then rotated into a lateral position to allow confirmation of the depth. A contralateral oblique view can often be utilized to better visualize the spinal needle as it approaches the spinolaminar line.

10. Now, based on the practitioner's preference, a loss of resistance (using air or saline) technique can be utilized to identify entrance into the epidural space. The needle stylet is removed and a syringe (either plastic or glass) with either saline or air is attached to the hub of the needle.

11. The needle is stabilized by holding the wings and advanced slowly in the same trajectory and the "loss of resistance" is checked by gently tapping on the syringe plunger. Once the loss of resistance has occurred, the advancement of the needle should be stopped to prevent a "wet tap" or spinal cord injury. Needle advancement should be stopped if the patient develops severe pain or paresthesias. Make sure there is negative aspirate for air, cerebrospinal fluid, and blood.

12. A negative aspiration check should be performed to ensure the needle is not placed into a blood vessel or cerebrospinal fluid. Connect the extension tubing to the needle and under live fluoroscopy, confirmation of epidural space entrance is verified by injection of 0.5 mL to 2 mL of nonionic contrast to verify spread into the epidural space by obtaining both lateral and AP views.

13. Digital subtraction can also be utilized to ensure absence of vascular flow.

14. After contrast confirmation of entry into the epidural space is done, the injectant mixture of corticosteroids and anesthetic is slowly injected.

15. The stylet is then reinserted into the needle, and the needle is withdrawn slowly.

16. Place a gauze on the needle entry point and apply pressure if there is bleeding. Place the sterile dressing or bandage at needle entry point.

17. Observe the patient postprocedure to assure that there are no adverse reactions. Provide the patient with postprocedure care instructions.

- Examples:
    1. AP: (Figure 5.2)
    2. Lateral: (Figure 5.3)

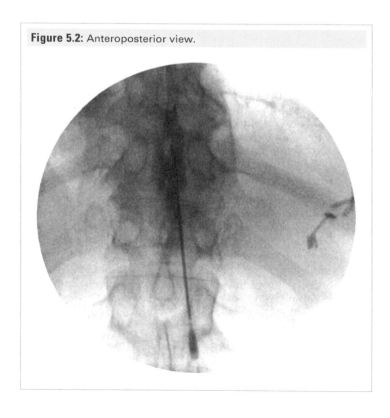

Figure 5.2: Anteroposterior view.

Figure 5.3: Lateral view.

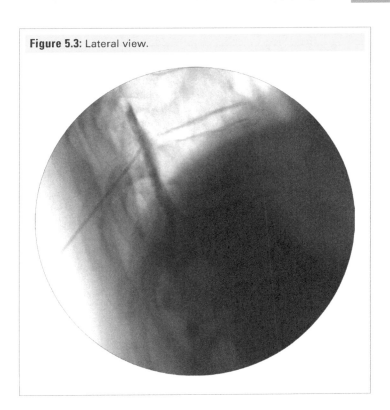

Sample Procedure Note

PREOPERATIVE DIAGNOSIS:	Thoracic radiculitis Thoracic disc displacement Thoracic spine pain
POSTOPERATIVE DIAGNOSIS:	Same
SURGEON:	＿＿＿
ASSISTANT:	＿＿＿
TITLE OF PROCEDURE:	＿＿＿Thoracic epidural steroid injection under fluoroscopic guidance

(continued)

(continued)

Thoracic epidurogram interpretation under fluoroscopic guidance

ANESTHESIA: Monitored anesthesia care
ESTIMATED BLOOD LOSS: None
COMPLICATIONS: None
DRAINS: None
IV Fluid ____mL lactated ringer

Indications: _____-year-old _____ (male/female) complaining of thoracic spine pain that radiates to the anterior chest wall. Our plan is to perform a thoracic epidural steroid injection under fluoroscopic guidance today. The risks and benefits of _____ thoracic epidural steroid injection were discussed in detail. The patient understands and accepts that the risks include, but are not limited to, increase in pain, nerve injury, infection, bleeding, hematoma, paralysis, spinal headache, stroke, discitis, and death. Alternatives to nerve blocks, or noninterventional therapy, were discussed and informed consent obtained.

DESCRIPTION OF PROCEDURE
Intravenous access was established. The patient was escorted to the fluoroscopy suite and placed in the prone position. Noninvasive monitoring was applied. Universal Site and Side Protocol was followed and documented. Safe Injection and Infection Control Practices as recommended by the Center for Disease Control, including the use of a face mask, were strictly followed. The thoracic area is widely prepped using _____ per protocol, and sterile drapes applied. Time out was performed. Using fluoroscopic guidance the thoracic vertebral bodies were identified. Using a 25-gauge needle, a skin wheal was raised with 1% lidocaine. Under fluoroscopic guidance in the AP and lateral views, an 18-gauge modified winged Tuohy needle was placed at the _____ interspace. The Tuohy needle was carried down to the epidural space using intermittent loss of resistance technique with saline to identify the epidural space. Once the epidural space was identified, AP and lateral projections of the fluoroscope

(continued)

(continued)

confirmed adequate needle placement. At this point, 2 mL of Omnipaque-240 contrast was injected under live fluoroscopic guidance through a T-connector extension tubing outlining a positive epidurogram. There was no evidence of intrathecal or intravascular spread. After negative aspiration for heme and CSF, 40 mg of Kenalog was injected with _____ mL of preservative-free _____ Marcaine through a T-connector extension tubing without complication. Once the procedure was completed, all needles were withdrawn from the patient intact. A bandage was applied to the puncture site. The patient tolerated this procedure well, there were no complications noted. The patient was discharged in hemodynamically and neurologically stable condition, with review of postprocedural instructions.

Plan: If the patient received 50% or greater improvement of their pain, we will repeat the procedure in 2 to 4 weeks' time. If today's injection does not alleviate the patient's pain by 50%, we will perform a diagnostic thoracic medial branch block under fluoroscopic guidance in 2 to 3 weeks.

_____

Attending Physician

INTERCOSTAL NERVE BLOCK

INDICATIONS: Chest wall pain syndrome, postthoracotomy syndrome, postherpetic neuralgia, costochondral joint dislocation, postmastectomy pain, shingles pain and acute herpes zoster, rib fractures, cancer-related pain of chest wall, neuropathic chest and upper abdominal pain

CONTRAINDICATIONS

- Patients in respiratory distress, history of pneumonectomy on the side of the planned procedure, patients on noninvasive positive pressure ventilation, patients with unknown rib dissection

RELEVANT ANATOMY

- The nerves enter the intercostal space after leaving the paravertebral space and lie in between the intercostal muscle and the pleura.

- Lateral to the paravertebral muscles, the prominent angles of the ribs are palpable as the primary landmark for intercostal nerve block.

- At the angle of the rib, the nerve lies between the innermost intercostal muscle and the inner intercostal muscle. Also, at this location, the thickness of the rib is 8 mm and the costal groove is known to be the widest.

- The intercostal nerves lie caudal to the intercostal vein and artery, on the inferior portion of the rib (vein–artery–nerve configuration) (Figure 5.4).

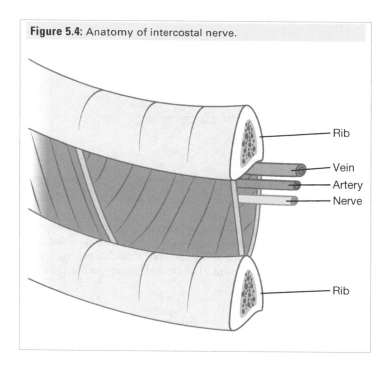

Figure 5.4: Anatomy of intercostal nerve.

Rib

Vein

Artery

Nerve

Rib

- The intercostal nerves are the primary rami of thoracic nerves T1 to T11.
- Most of the T1 nerve fibers combine with C8 to form the lower trunk of the brachial plexus.

PATIENT POSITION

- Place patient in prone position
- Place pillow under the abdomen and allow both upper extremities to hang over the sides of the fluoroscopy table.

TECHNIQUE

- Prep the skin using a chlorhexidine prep (preferably), povidone iodine, or isopropyl alcohol are all options for antiseptic agents for use in percutaneous spine procedures.
- Place the C-arm in the AP view, confirm the target level. Tilting of the C-arm caudal or cranial may be required to obtain a true AP image.
- The target needle end point is the inferior border of the corresponding level. The target entry point is at 3 cm to 4 cm from midline and inferior border of the targeted rib.
- Infiltrate the skin and subcutaneous tissues with 3 mL to 5 mL of 1% lidocaine using a 25- or 27-gauge needle.
- Using a 22-gauge curved Quincke spinal needle, direct the needle to the inferior border of the rib parallel to the C-arm beam.
- Once the needle touches the os of the inferior border of the rib, the needle can be slowly walked off in the caudal direction until it slips off the inferior rib margin.
- Obtain AP and lateral projection to confirm adequate depth.
- Perform a negative aspiration check.
- Inject contrast to ensure no intravascular spread.
- Inject the combination of steroid and anesthetic.
- Withdraw needles from the patient.
- Example:
  1. AP: (Figure 5.5)

Figure 5.5: Anteroposterior view.

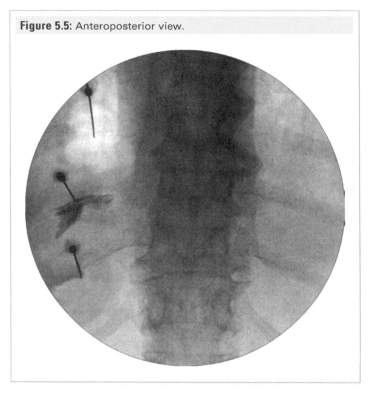

Sample Procedure Note

PREOPERATIVE DIAGNOSIS:	Intercostal neuralgia Other nerve root plexus disorder Thoracic spine pain
POSTOPERATIVE DIAGNOSIS:	Same
SURGEON:	____
ASSISTANT:	____
TITLE OF PROCEDURE:	____Intercostal nerve block under fluoroscopic guidance (**Video 5.1**)

https://bcove.video/2IkZVSo

(continued)

(continued)

ANESTHESIA: Monitored anesthesia care
ESTIMATED BLOOD LOSS: None
COMPLICATIONS: None
DRAINS: None
IV FLUID   _____ mL Lactated
                               Ringer

Indications: _____-year-old _____ (male/female) complaining of thoracic spine and flank pain that radiates to the anterior chest wall. Our plan is to perform an intercostal nerve block under fluoroscopic guidance today. The risks and benefits of _____ intercostal nerve block were discussed in detail. The patient understands and accepts that the risks include, but are not limited to, increase in pain, nerve injury, infection, bleeding, seizure, hematoma, paralysis, pneumothorax, stroke, and death. Alternatives to nerve blocks, or noninterventional therapy, were discussed and informed consent obtained.

DESCRIPTION OF PROCEDURE
Intravenous access was established. The patient was escorted to the fluoroscopy suite and placed in the prone position. Noninvasive monitoring was applied. Universal Site and Side Protocol was followed and documented. Safe Injection and Infection Control Practices as recommended by the Center for Disease Control, including the use of a face mask, were strictly followed. The thoracic area is widely prepped using _____ per protocol, and sterile drapes applied. Time out was performed. Using fluoroscopic guidance the thoracic vertebral bodies and ribs were identified. Using a 25-gauge needle, a skin wheal was raised with 1% lidocaine. Under fluoroscopic guidance in the AP view, a 22-gauge curved Quincke spinal needle was placed over the _____ rib on the _____ side 3 cm to 4 cm from the midline. The spinal needle was carried down until the rib was in contact. Once the rib was in contact, the needle was directed to the caudad direction until the needle tip slipped off of the bone. At this point, AP and lateral projections of the fluoroscope confirmed adequate needle placement. At this point, 2 mL of Omnipaque-240 contrast was injected under live fluoroscopic guidance through a T-connector extension tubing outlining a positive neurogram. There was no evidence of intravascular spread. After negative

---

(continued)

(*continued*)

aspiration for heme, 40 mg of Kenalog was injected with _____ mL of preservative-free _____ Marcaine in divided doses through a T-connector extension tubing without complication. Once the procedure was completed, all needles were withdrawn from the patient intact. A bandage was applied to the puncture site. The patient tolerated this procedure well, there were no complications noted. The patient was discharged in hemodynamically and neurologically stable condition, with review of postprocedural instructions.

Plan: If the patient received 50% or greater improvement of their pain, we will repeat the procedure in 2 to 4 weeks' time. If today's injection does not alleviate the patient's pain by 50%, we will perform a diagnostic thoracic medial branch block under fluoroscopic guidance in 2 to 3 weeks.

Attending Physician

Coding:

PROCEDURES	
Thoracic interlaminar epidural	62310
Thoracic transforaminal first level	64479
Thoracic transforaminal additional level	64480
Thoracic medial branch block or intra-articular facet joint injection first level	64490
Thoracic medial branch block or intra-articular facet joint injection second level	64491
Thoracic medial branch block or intra-articular facet joint injection third level	64492
Bilateral modifier	50
RFA—first thoracic level	64633
RFA additional levels	64634

(*continued*)

(*continued*)

Intercostal nerve injection (single level)	**64420**
Intercostal nerve injection (multiple levels)	**64421**
INJECTABLES	**J-codes**
Low osmolar contrast material (Omnipaque 300)	**Q9967**
Low osmolar contrast material (Omnipaque 240)	**Q9966**
Betamethasone (Celestone 3 mg)	**J0702**
Betamethasone (Celestone 4 mg)	**J0704**
Dexamethasone sodium phosphate 1 mg	**J1100**
Depo-Medrol (40 mg)	**J1030**
Depo-Medrol (80 mg)	**J1040**
Triamcinolone (per 10 mg)	**J3301**
Diphenhydramine (injection up to 50 mg)	**J1200**
Versed (per mg)	**J2250**
Fentanyl (0.1 mg)	**J3010**

RFA, radiofrequency ablation.

Video

 Video 5.1 Intercostal Nerve Block

https://bcove.video/2IkZVSo

Lumbar Spine

6

LUMBAR SPONDYLOSIS WITHOUT MYELOPATHY

DEFINITION: Normal aging degenerative process of the joints forming the spinal column: posteriorly, the zygapophysial joints and anteriorly the intervertebral disk. These degenerative changes occur with increasing age and may be associated with low back pain. If there is unstableness to the vertebrae that is degenerative, the amount of pain is greater. The pain from the degeneration often flows down to the buttock and thighs. In most cases, the pain is less severe and/or of no significance. If myelopathy is present, the spondylosis can lead to cauda equina compression.

EPIDEMIOLOGY: The lifetime incidence of low back pain is between 60% and 90% of the population. Lumbar spondylosis is uncommon in the first three decades of life. In patients with low back pain, the prevalence of lumbar spondylosis ranges from 10% to 75%, depending on the diagnostic criteria.

RISK FACTORS: The exact cause of disk degeneration is unknown; however, previous back injury leading to an annular tear, obesity, female gender, heavy regular exercises that stresses the disk and annular ligament (crossfit), occupations requiring repeat lifting, patients with previous history of lumbar surgery have changes in lumbar biomechanics, joint overload from malalignment, abnormal facet joint orientation, changes of increasing age (osteophyte formation, advanced cartilage changes, and subchondral sclerosis).

COMPLICATIONS: Due to the osteophyte formation and disc desiccation the facet joints are hypertrophied. This may lead to an intervertebral foramen or spinal canal narrowing. These changes may result in central or lateral stenosis, radiculopathy, and in severe cases, cauda equina syndrome.

THE DEGENERATIVE CASCADE OF SPONDYLOSIS PROPOSED BY KIRKALDY-WILLIS AND BERNARD	
Phase I: Dysfunction Phase	• Initial effects of repetitive microtrauma with development of circumferential painful tears of the outer, innervated annulus • End-plate separation that may compromise the disc nutritional supply and waste removal • Fissure development by vascular tissue and nerve endings, increasing the innervation and the disc's ability for pain signal transmission
Phase II: Instability Phase	• Loss of mechanical integrity which leads to continuous disc changes of resorption, internal disruption, and annular tears (high-intensity zone), combined with continuous zygapophyseal degeneration may cause further subluxation and instability
Phase III: Stabilization Phase	• Continuation of disc space narrowing • Fibrosis development • Formation of osteophytes and transdiscal bridging • Lumbar spinal stenosis occurs at the end stage of spondylosis

ASSESSMENT

i. Symptoms of lumbar spondylosis can be acute or gradual onset. Pain may be referred unilaterally or bilaterally to the buttock, hip, groin, and thigh regions.

ii. Pain is typically worse with extension, rotation, and standing. Pain is generally alleviated by lying or lumbar spine forward flexion.

iii. Patients may notice a strange sensation such as pins and needles with numbness of the affected lower extremity.

iv. Lumbar spondylosis without myelopathy should not exhibit neurologic symptoms. If myelopathy is suspected, assessment of objective weakness, balance deficits, gait abnormalities, and bowel/bladder function should be done.

v. Back pain following infection or a history of malignancy may suggest more serious conditions.

PHYSICAL EXAMINATION

i. Inspection: Evaluation of paraspinal muscles (fullness, asymmetry, and atrophy). Assess for flattening of lumbar lordotic curves and rotation or lateral bending at the thoracolumbar area and sacroiliac joint.

ii. Palpation: Palpate along the lumbar paraspinals to localize and reproduce any point tenderness, which may be present with facet arthropathy.

iii. Range of motion: Assess through lumbar flexion, extension, lateral bending bilaterally and rotation bilaterally.

iv. Muscle strength should be performed to determine if objective or pain-limited weakness is present and if it corresponds to single root, multiple roots, or peripheral nerve or lumbosacral plexus.

v. Due to the pain distribution overlapping other diagnosis, evaluation of the hip and sacroiliac joint should be performed routinely.

vi. Special tests:

1. Kemp's test: Provocative test to detect pain from the lumbar spine facet joints. Performed by stabilizing the lumbar spine with one hand and supporting the patient's contralateral shoulder with the other hand. Advise patient to lean away from the examiner, then twist the torso into forward flexion and eventually return back into the lateral flexion and extension.

DIAGNOSTIC TESTS

i. Imaging may be performed to rule out other disorder. X-ray, MRI, and CT scan are performed for the evaluation of facet joints.

ii. X-rays are not sufficiently sensitive for detecting early facet arthropathy. Lateral views are recommended to study alignment and the presence of spondylolisthesis.

TABLE 6.1: INNERVATION OF LUMBAR FACET JOINTS

FACET JOINT	INNERVATION
L2–L3	L1–L2 medial branches
L3–L4	L2 and L3 medial branches
L4–L5	L3 and L4 medial branches
L5–S1	L4 medial branch and L5 dorsal ramus

iii. MRI is not necessary but may allow evaluation of soft tissues and neural elements and synovial fluid in facet joints. A CT scan may be performed if MRI is inaccessible.

TREATMENT

i. Treatment of acute low back pain which has been occurring for less than 6 weeks includes physical therapy.

ii. Taking supine breaks may be helpful.

iii. Depending on severity of the low back pain, use of acetaminophen/nonsteroidal anti-inflammatory drugs (NSAIDs) may be beneficial.

iv. If the patient reports muscle spasms with pain, use of muscle relaxants and modalities such as heat, transcutaneous electrical nerve stimulation (TENS) units, and massage may be helpful.

v. Triggering activities should be avoided.

vi. Diagnostic and/or therapeutic medial branch blocks may be performed to confirm the diagnosis. A radiofrequency ablation of the medial branches may be performed after one or two successful diagnostic medial branch blocks (see Table 6.1).

LUMBOSACRAL RADICULOPATHY

DEFINITION: Lumbosacral radiculopathy is defined as the dysfunction of a spinal nerve root emerging from the level of the lumbosacral spine. It is commonly associated with a disc herniation. It usually presents with pain, numbness, reflex changes, and/or weakness in a specific radicular pattern. It has a variable presence of weakness, changes in the reflexes, and development of paresthesias leading to interferences of activities of daily living (ADLs).

RISK FACTORS: Lumbar radiculopathy is usually secondary to compression associated with an inflammatory process causing injury to a spinal nerve or nerve root. Other causes of lumbar radiculopathy may also be secondary to a herniated disk, foraminal stenosis, osteophyte formation, or another cause of compression of the spinal nerve. Rare causes of secondary lumbar radiculopathy include etiologies from infectious process, rheumatologic conditions, neurological conditions, and musculoskeletal injuries.

EPIDEMIOLOGY: The prevalence of lumbosacral radiculopathy is estimated to be approximately 3% to 5%. It is distributed equally in men and women. Men in their 40s are most likely to develop symptoms of radiculopathy whereas women are commonly affected between ages 50 and 60. Degenerative spondyloarthropathies are the most common cause.

COMPLICATIONS: Cauda equina syndrome is a surgical emergency that is described as an extreme pressure and swelling of the group of nerves at the end of the spinal cord. This results in a characteristic pattern of pain, numbness, and tingling in addition to urogenital symptoms. Cauda equina syndrome complications can result in permanent paralysis, impaired bladder or bowel control, and difficulty in ambulation. Single root radicular symptoms with weakness that is worsening overtime is another complication of lumbar radiculopathy and should be treated with urgent surgical treatment.

ASSESSMENT

i. Patients who are suffering from lumbar radiculopathy note sharp pain, paresthesias, tingling, and numbness in the distribution of the nerve root or roots that are affected. Limb pain and paresthesias dominate while back pain is also usually present. The limb pain paresthesias may fit a specific dermatomal distribution. Decreased sensation, weakness, and reflex changes may be seen on physical examination.

■ Rule out red flag symptoms to rule out tumor, infection, or cauda equina.

a. Red flags in spinal pain indicate that there may be a serious or life-threatening cause of back pain and will require further workup.

INFECTION	MALIGNANCY (METASTASIS)	CAUDA EQUINA
• History of IV drug abuse • Recent spine surgery within the last 12 months • Fever and chills • Recent bacterial infection (wounds, lung, skin, UTI, pyelonephritis) • Immuno-compromised	• Weight loss • Pain worse at night or at rest • Prior history of cancer	• Saddle anesthesia • Urine incontinence • Fecal incontinence • Decreased anal sphincter tone • Worsening of weakness and numbness • Progressive neurological deficits

IV, intravenous; UTI, urinary tract infection.

ii. Physical examination:

1. Inspection: Check alignment, prior surgical scars, muscle atrophy, or skin defects.

2. Palpation: Assess for local tenderness of the spinous processes, cervical, thoracic, or lumbar paraspinal atrophy and asymmetry.

3. Range of motion: Document range of motion (ROM) in forward flexion, hyperextension, rotation bilaterally, lateral bending bilaterally.

4. Special tests:

   a. Straight leg raise test (Lasègue test or Lazarević's sign): Patient lies supine and then raises the ipsilateral leg with the knee extended. If pain is reproduced at 30 to 70 degrees, L4–S1 spinal nerve root pathology or radiculopathy as the source of pain is likely. Symptoms may exacerbate by adding ankle dorsiflexion to the straight leg raise test, adding more sensitivity to the test. Pain produced at less than 30 degrees of hip flexion might indicate acute spondylolisthesis, disc protrusion or extrusion, acute dural inflammation, or somatization. Pain produced at greater than 70 degrees of hip flexion might indicate tightness of the hamstrings, gluteus maximus, or sacroiliac joint or hip pathology.

HERNIATION	COMMON LUMBAR ROOT AFFECTED	PAIN	SENSORY CHANGES	WEAKNESS	REFLEX CHANGES
L3–L4	L4	Low back, shin, thigh, and leg	Shin numbness	Knee extensors and ankle dorsiflexors	Knee jerk absent

(continued)

(continued)

HERNIATION	COMMON LUMBAR ROOT AFFECTED	PAIN	SENSORY CHANGES	WEAKNESS	REFLEX CHANGES
L4-L5	L5	Low back, posterior thigh, and leg	Numbness on the dorsum of foot, and first web space	Extensor hallucis longus	

(continued)

(continued)

L5–S1	S1	Low back, posterior calf, and leg	Numbness of lateral foot	Gastrocnemius and soleus	Ankle jerk absent

b. Reverse straight leg raise test (femoral nerve stretch test): Patient lies in prone or lateral decubitus position, then the patient's knee is maximally flexed while the hip is extended. A positive test involves pain in the L2, L3, or L4 nerve root.

c. Crossed straight leg raise test: Patient lies supine and then raises the unaffected leg with the knee extended. Positive when radicular pain occurs in the affected extremity.

d. Hoover's sign: Test to exclude organic from nonorganic paresis of the leg. The test is performed by placing both examiner's hands under the patient's heels while the patient is supine. Then, ask the patient to raise one leg. If the examiner cannot feel the downward pressure in the resting leg, the patient is not likely giving honest effort. If the patient is making an honest effort, the examiner should feel the resting heel pushing down against the examiner's hand.

5. Diagnostic tests:

a. Imaging: Usually indicated if symptoms present for more than 1 month, unless progressive neurologic functional deficits are present, or red flags described earlier. Usually, plain radiographs are the first-line imaging modality ordered. Often, initial plain radiographs are not helpful in establishing a diagnosis in younger patients. X-rays may also be useful in documenting abnormal curvature of the spine, evaluation and grading of spondylolisthesis, and screen for fractures. Lumbar MRI is often used as a confirmatory test of the clinical diagnosis. Often, up to 36% of asymptomatic adults have disc herniations on lumbar MRI. Consider a lumbar CT scan or CT myelogram if MRI is contraindicated.

b. Nerve conduction studies (NCS) and electromyography (EMG) may be performed to distinguish which nerve root(s) may be affected. NCS may show decreased amplitude or normal responses. EMG is more diagnostic, and shows spontaneous potential, abnormal insertional activity such as positive sharp waves and fibrillation potentials. EMG testing of the lumbar paraspinal muscles is very sensitive for lumbar radiculopathy and/or myelopathy. EMG is usually negative for pathology for the first 3 to 4 weeks after symptom onset, and should not be ordered unless symptom onset is greater than 4 weeks.

  c. Electrodiagnostic protocol for lumbar radiculopathy:

    i. NCS: Minimum of one motor NCS and one sensory NCS in the symptomatic extremity to determine if other concomitant nerve disorder is present. Sensory nerve action potentials (SNAPs) should be normal in radiculopathy.

      1. Include tibial and fibular compound muscle action potentials (CMAPs) and sural SNAPs.

      2. CMAP/SNAP of other nerves if 1 + NCS is found to be abnormal or peripheral neuropathy is suspected. Consider NCS of upper extremity if a polyneuropathy is suspected.

      3. H-reflex for tibial nerve may be performed if S1 radiculopathy is suspected. H reflex may be decreased or absent in a S1 radiculopathy.

    ii. EMG:

      1. Test five or more muscles in the symptomatic side covering all myotomes +/− paraspinals of the suspected spinal level.

      2. Test one to two muscles innervated by the suspected root level and different peripheral nerves.

      3. If a muscle is abnormal, consider testing the contralateral muscle.

    iii. Recommended EMG muscles (see following table)

6. Treatment

  a. Treatment protocol includes reduction of inflammation by avoidance of bending and lifting which causes increased intradiscal pressure. NSAIDs are often used on an as needed basis. Antineuropathic agents (gabapentin, lamotrigine, and amitriptyline) are also used for nerve stabilization.

  b. Mild cases may be treated with NSAIDs, Tylenol, and topical medications.

  c. Medrol dose pack may be required for acute phases.

  d. Muscle relaxants and opiates may be used in refractory cases.

MUSCLE	NERVE	L2	L3	L4	L5	S1	S2
Iliopsoas	Femoral nerve	+	+				
Vastus medialis	Femoral nerve		+	+			
Tibialis anterior	Deep fibular nerve			+	+		
Extensor hallucis longus	Deep fibular nerve				+	+	
Bicep femoris long head	Sciatic nerve (tibial portion)				+	+	
Bicep femoris short head	Sciatic nerve (fibular portion)				+	+	
Medial gastrocnemius	Tibial nerve				+	+	+
Tensor fasciae latae	Superior gluteal nerve				+	+	
Gluteus medius	Superior gluteal nerve				+	+	
Gluteus maximus	Inferior gluteal nerve				+	+	
Piriformis	Nerve to piriformis				+	+	+
Abductor hallucis	Tibial nerve					+	+

e. Selective nerve root blocks, paravertebral blocks, epidural steroid injections may be used during acute or subacute lumbar radiculopathy.

f. Chronic pain management includes the following:

　　i. NSAIDs

　　ii. Gabapentin/pregabalin

　　iii. Tricyclic antidepressants (TCAs)

　　iv. Anxiolytics

　　v. Compound creams

g. Use of muscle relaxants should be used in patients with spasms or spasticity.

h. Use of opioid analgesics should be limited in chronic pain management.

i. If chronic pain is significantly interfering with sleep and activities of daily living, an interdisciplinary approach should be implemented.

7. Rehabilitation program:

a. Goal: pain reduction, functional improvement, increase pain-free ROM, increase back and core stability.

b. General stretching programs, foraminal opening maneuvers. A McKenzie Method Assessment may be prescribed.

c. Modalities: ice, heat, TENS units, massage, and electrical stimulation.

d. Progressive stretching in full ROM of lumbar spine.

e. Strengthening of core muscles (paraspinals, glutes, and abdominal muscles)

f. Development of a home exercise regimen.

8. Interdisciplinary coordination of care:

a. Surgery (orthopedic or neurosurgery), psychology, psychiatry, support groups, physical and occupational therapies may all play a role.

b. Infectious disease, oncology, urology, and plastic surgery may also play a role depending on the etiology and severity of the condition.

LUMBAR SPINAL STENOSIS

DEFINITION: Lumbar spinal stenosis is defined as narrowing of the central (intraspinal) canal, narrowing of the neural foramen, or narrowing of the lateral recess. Compression of the nerve roots may lead to ischemia and inflammation causing neurogenic claudication. The syndrome causes symptoms characterized as neurogenic claudication, progressive paresthesia, and pain with ambulation. Symptoms are often relieved by sitting or leaning forward.

RISK FACTORS: Spondylosis (degenerative joint disease) is the result of osteoarthritic changes in the spine. It is the most common cause of spinal stenosis and typically affects individuals older than 60 years. Weight gain has also been known to be a contributing factor. Trauma, wear and tear, along with other lifestyle factors lead to loss of disc height, disc protrusion, and loading of the posterior elements of the spine, including the zygapophyseal joints (facet joints). The facet joint arthropathy, ligamentum flavum hypertrophy, and development of osteophytes also occur as the degenerative process progresses. This degenerative process then can infiltrate on the central canal and the neural foramina. Other causes include ankylosing spondylitis, Paget's disease, diffuse idiopathic skeletal hyperostosis (DISH), rheumatoid arthritis, and congenital malformation such as spina bifida, achondroplasia, and myelomeningocele. Space-occupying lesions such as tumors, synovial cysts, neural cysts, lipomas, and epidural lipomatosis may also cause neuroforaminal stenosis.

A normal adult lumbar spinal canal diameter is 15 mm to 27 mm.

i. A central lumbar spinal stenosis occurs when this diameter is less than 12 mm.

ii. A lateral foraminal stenosis occurs when there is less than 3 mm to 4 mm between the superior articular process and posterior vertebral margin.

Complications include cauda equina syndrome, which is characterized by significant bilateral lower extremities weakness, bowel and bladder dysfunction, saddle anesthesia, and erectile dysfunction. This is a surgical emergency that may require immediate decompression in the attempt to delay possible long-term neurological dysfunction.

ASSESSMENT

i. Patients usually experience a progressive increase in pain over many years. During the pain cycle, the distribution of the pain changes involves the buttocks and/or bilateral lower extremities. The Classical indication of lumbar spinal stenosis is the presence of "neurogenic claudication." Neurogenic claudication is defined as the development of pain in one or both lower extremities upon walking, typically downhill. The patient describes that the pain starts centrally and moves toward the lower extremities as the patient continues to walk. In contrast, vascular claudication is described as pain starting in the periphery and radiating toward the back. The patient may give a history of adopting a flexed position to prevent pain with prolonged standing. They may ambulate with a prominent forward lumbar flexion, commonly described as Simian gait or "shopping cart sign." Patients describe the quality of the pain to resemble symptoms seen in osteoarthritis; achy, stiffness, weather-related initially. Lateral recess, subarticular, or a foraminal stenosis may present with a unilateral radiculopathy.

ii. Physical examination:

1. Range of motion of the lumbar spine is limited likely secondary to a degenerative process within the lumbar spine. Typically, there is a limited extension of the lumbar spine when compared to lumbar forward flexion. Often, if the lumbar hyperextension is maintained for greater than 30 seconds, it may produce leg symptoms.

2. Palpation of the lumbar spine should be performed but does not usually reproduce the patient's pain. However, it is helpful to rule out a red flag diagnosis.

3. A straight leg raise may reproduce pain if the patient is suffering from a disk herniation as well.

4. L5 nerve root is most frequently affected, thus there may be associated weakness in muscles innervated by L5 nerve root (e.g., tibialis anterior and/or extensor hallucis longus).

5. Sensory examination may reveal changes, especially in the L4L5 dermatomes.

6. The ankle and/or knee jerks may be diminished or absent.

7. Functional assessment includes assessment of gait, balance (Romberg test), and pain while seated.

8. Special tests:

   a. Straight leg raise test (Lasègue test or Lazarević's sign): Patient lies supine and then raises the ipsilateral leg with the knee extended. If pain is reproduced at 30 to 70 degrees, L4S1 spinal nerve root pathology or radiculopathy as the source of pain is likely. Symptoms may be exacerbated by adding ankle dorsiflexion to the straight leg raise test, adding more sensitivity to the test. Pain produced at less than 30 degrees of hip flexion might indicate acute spondylolisthesis, disc protrusion or extrusion, acute dural inflammation, or somatization. Pain produced at greater than 70 degrees of hip flexion might indicate tightness of the hamstrings, gluteus maximus, or sacroiliac joint or hip pathology.

   b. Seated slump test: The patient is seated with hands behind the back to position the spine in neutral. Next, have the patient slump forward at the thoracic and lumbar spine. If this does not reproduce the patient's pain, have the patient flex the neck by placing the patient's chin on the test, and extending the knee. If knee extension reproduces the pain, have the patient extend the neck position to neutral. If the patient is still unable to extend his or her knee, the test is considered positive. If knee extension does not reproduce the patient's pain, have the patient dorsiflex the ankle. If the pain is reproduced with ankle dorsiflexion, then also the test is considered positive.

   c. Kemp's test: Provocative test to detect pain from the lumbar spine facet joints. Performed by stabilizing the lumbar spine with one hand and supporting the patient's contralateral shoulder with the other hand. Advise patient to lean away from the examiner, then twist the torso into forward flexion and eventually returned back into the lateral flexion and extension.

   d. Femoral nerve stretch test: Patient lies in prone or lateral decubitus position, and then the patient's knee is maximally flexed while the hip is extended. A positive test involves pain in the L2, L3, or L4 nerve root.

iii. Diagnostic tests:

   1. There are no objective standards for the clinical diagnosis of lumbar spinal stenosis. Lumbar spinal stenosis syndrome

is typically diagnosed by utilization of history, physical examination, and imaging.

2. Imaging:

    a. Plain x-ray films may reveal evidence of spondylolisthesis, disc space narrowing, marginal osteophyte development, facet arthropathy, vertebral endplate changes, foraminal narrowing, and so on.

    b. MRI is thought to be the gold standard because it allows visualization of bone and soft-tissue anatomy. A normal adult lumbar spinal canal diameter is 15 mm to 27 mm. Lumbar spinal stenosis results when this diameter is less than 12 mm.

        i. Relative lumbar spinal stenosis: 10 mm to 12 mm

        ii. Absolute lumbar spinal stenosis: less than 10 mm

3. HLA-B27 and serum protein electrophoresis (SPEP) may be ordered if ankylosing spondylitis and multiple myeloma is suspected.

iv. Treatment:

1. Treatment is usually conservative for pain if no myelopathic symptoms are present. NSAIDs and Tylenol may be used at regular intervals. A short course of opioids and/or muscle relaxants may be used in more severe cases.

2. Steroid packs may be used in patients with functionally limiting pain with a 7- to 10-day steroid taper.

3. Neuropathic pain medications may be used for patients with radicular pain. Gabapentin, pregabalin, and TCAs are usually first-line agents.

4. An epidural steroid injection (interlaminar, caudal, or transforaminal approaches) under fluoroscopic guidance is suggested to provide short-term symptomatic relief (2 weeks to 6 months) depending on severity of symptoms.

v. Rehabilitation program:

1. Goal: pain reduction, functional improvement, increase pain-free ROM

2. Modalities: ice, heat, TENS, massage, E-stim

3. A lumbar stabilization program may be prescribed with a focus on flexion-biased exercises (Williams exercises), pelvic posture correction, core strengthening, to prevent

excessive lumbar extension and to emphasize hamstring relaxation.

a. These therapeutic exercises include hip flexor, hamstring, lumbar paraspinal stretching, abdominal and gluteal strengthening exercises such as pelvic tilts, trunk raises, and bridging.

b. Conditioning exercises such as inclined treadmill, stationary bicycle, and aquatic exercises

c. Avoidance of exercises that may put nerve roots under excessive tension

4. Development of a home exercise program

LUMBAR SPONDYLOLISTHESIS

DEFINITION: Spondylolisthesis is a condition where one vertebral body displaces anteriorly or posteriorly with respect to an adjacent vertebral body, causing worsening of the spinal canal narrowing. The most commonly involved levels are L4L5, L5S1, and L3L4. The pars interarticularis may be fractured due to these degenerative changes causing instability, and vertebral body displacement.

i. Meyerding classification (Figure 6.1) is used to grade the severity of spondylolisthesis. Severity is rated by the percentage of slippage of the posterior edge of the vertebral body above the superior surface of the vertebral body below.

1. Grade I: 0% to 25%

2. Grade II: 26% to 50%

3. Grade III: 51% to 75%

4. Grade IV: 76% to 100%

5. Although it is technically not a part of the Meyerding spondylolisthesis grading scale, some clinicians use grade 5 to diagnose cases in which a vertebra has slipped completely off the vertebra below it. This condition is also known as spondyloptosis. Grade V (spondyloptosis): greater than 100%

RISK FACTORS

i. Genetic predisposition, individuals with high physical stress, repetitive lumbar extension, sports such as gymnastics, diving, weight lifting, wrestling, acrobatics, and football.

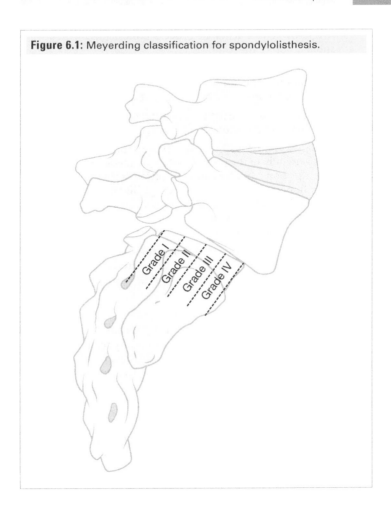

Figure 6.1: Meyerding classification for spondylolisthesis.

ETIOLOGY

i. Lytic isthmic spondylolisthesis: pars interarticularis stress fracture; commonly occurs at L5S1; most common form of spondylolisthesis. Normally develops in children aged 5 to 15; often causing no symptoms. The slippage of the vertebra normally does not progress.

ii. Degenerative spondylolisthesis: also a common form of spondylolisthesis that presents as a normal aging process due to prevalence of arthritis in the elderly. Presence of chronic facet arthropathy causes articular process remodeling, which leads to subluxation of the joint.

iii. Dysplastic spondylolisthesis: rare congenital defect from the malformation of the lumbosacral junction; specifically the facet joints are underdeveloped or presence of spina bifida from birth.

iv. Traumatic spondylolisthesis: fracture of the inferior facets, pedicle, pars interarticularis, or posterior elements.

v. Pathologic spondylolisthesis: rare type of spondylolisthesis that occurs generally in the presence of a rare metabolic disease that affects the bone (malignancy, infection, osteoporosis, osteogenesis imperfecta, or collagen storage diseases, etc.). Damage occurs to the posterior elements. Other causes include primary or metastatic cancer or infection that disrupts the integrity of the posterior elements.

vi. Congenital: rare, however rapidly progressive. It is associated with severe neurological deficits. Characterized by malformation of the lumbosacral junction and facet joints.

COMPLICATIONS

i. Cauda equina syndrome can be a significant complication of lumbar spondylolisthesis. This is commonly seen in degenerative spondylolisthesis. Assessment of bowel and bladder function, saddle anesthesia, or genital organ dysfunction should be performed.

ASSESSMENT

i. Most individuals with lumbar spondylolisthesis are asymptomatic. Patients who do develop symptoms present with diffuse and dull low back pain, leg pain, or combination. Patients complain of back pain with activity and are relieved with lying recumbent. The leg pain numbness and tingling is described predominantly in a dermatomal distribution if the nerve is being compressed in the lateral recess at the level of the pars interarticularis defect. Spondylolysis is one of the most common causes of back pain in children. A detailed assessment should be performed if a traumatic incident or sports-related injury is suspected. History should include evaluation of stool and urinary incontinence, weakness, or sexual dysfunction.

ii. Physical examination:

1. Inspection may reveal an increased lumbar lordosis, postural changes, and/or flattening of the buttocks.

2. Palpation of the spine may illicit midline tenderness, and a step-off of the spinous process may be felt above the level of the slip. This is a specific finding with grades 3 and more.

3. Range of motion may be difficult due to limited flexion of the lumbar spine due to paraspinal spasms. Paraspinals attempt to prevent shear forces across the affected lumbar segment.

4. Focal weakness, sensory loss may be evident secondary the degree of nerve compression in the lateral recess.

5. Dural tension signs are typically negative.

6. Hamstring contractures may be evident in children.

7. If cauda equina syndrome is suspected, a rectal exam for sensation and tone should be performed.

8. Gait assessment may reveal a waddling gait due to increased pelvic rotation, tight hamstrings, and increased lumbar lordosis from compensation.

iii. Diagnostic tests:

1. Initial plain radiographic evaluation is appropriate, which should consist of anteroposterior (AP) and lateral flexion–extension radiographics. A standing and supine lateral radiograph is also important to evaluate for a translational instability. An oblique view may allow better visualization of a pars interarticularis fracture.

2. CT scan will better provide bony details of pathology, and an MRI will give better visualization of the soft-tissue abnormalities such as compression of dural sac.

3. Bone scans and single-photon emission CT (SPECT) scans are used for determining if the defect is acute or chronic.

iv. Treatment:

1. Activity modification: relative rest and avoidance of hyperextension

2. Medications: NSAIDs, acetaminophen, short course of opioids for breakthrough pain. Short course of oral

steroids and neuropathic agents if radiculopathy is suspected.

3. Thoracolumbosacral (TLSO) brace: for acute spondylolysis in children and young adults, a rigid antilordotic thoracolumbosacral orthosis has been suggested to use for up to 5 to 6 months.

4. Procedures: Transforaminal or interlaminar epidural steroid injections may be beneficial if radicular symptoms are present. Medial branch blocks may also be beneficial if facet mediated axial pain.

5. Surgical consultation may be warranted in cases involving neurologic deficits, or presence of cauda equina syndrome.

v. Rehabilitation program:

1. Goal: alleviate pain; increase core stability

2. Modalities: thermal treatments, electrical stimulation, lumbar traction

3. Stretching: hamstring and quadriceps stretching

4. Strengthening program for spinal stabilizers for lumbar flexion (hip flexors, abdominals, lumbar paraspinals)

POSTLAMINECTOMY PAIN

DEFINITION: Also known as failed back surgery syndrome; used to describe persistent or recurrent low back pain, with or without lower extremity symptoms following one or more spine surgeries. Thus, the outcome of the lumbar spinal surgery does not meet the presurgical expectations of patient or physician.

RISK FACTORS

i. Preoperative factors:

1. Patient: poor coping strategies, anxiety, depression, pain sensitization and magnification, hypochondriasis, litigation, worker's compensation, and development of myofascial pain syndrome, history of smoking, diabetes, and other causes which may lead to poor healing postoperatively

2. Surgical: candidate selection, revision surgery, (approximately 50% increase in risk in spinal instability with greater than four revision), surgery technique selection

ii. Intraoperative factors: inadequate lateral recess decompression, incorrect level of surgery

iii. Postoperative factors: development of epidural fibrosis leading to tethering effect, inadequate nutrition, disruption of vascular supply to nerve root, surgical complications, (nerve injury, infection, hematoma development), and progressive multisegmental spinal stenosis, development of cauda equina syndrome

ETIOLOGY: Typically, the intrinsic features of the pain experienced by patients with postlaminectomy syndrome are consistent with the underlying pathology. A variety of postlaminectomy pain is neuropathic pain, which is caused initially by primary injury to the nervous system. In patients with postlaminectomy syndrome, the initial spinal disorder that caused the nerve injury prior to surgery may cause neuropathic pain to return. Another variety of pain that may persist after back surgery is radicular pain that travels along the dermatome or sensory distribution of a nerve due to an inflammatory process or irritation of the nerve root. First, nerve root irritation may arise from a spinal disc bulge, herniation, or annular tear. Finally, neuropathic and radicular pain can result in central sensitization of nervous tissues, or harmful changes to pain receptors.

EPIDEMIOLOGY

i. There are approximately more than 1 million spinal surgeries performed. The incidence of postlaminectomy syndrome is estimated to be between 11% and 40% and is dependent on the type of surgery performed.

ASSESSMENT

i. History:

1. History should include the location and pattern of pain, description of the quality and aggravating and alleviating factors. The location of the low back versus leg can help differentiate the etiology. Prior pain treatments (pharmacological, nonpharmacological, interventional, and surgical treatment), their timeline along with their efficacy should be assessed and evaluated.

ii. Physical Examination:

1. Focused spinal physical examination should include observation of surgical scars, posture, alignment of the spine, gait, and balance. Spine ROM should also be evaluated.

2. Special tests include testing for nerve root impingement signs such as straight leg raise, seated slump test, and femoral nerve stretch test should be performed as well.

3. A functional assessment may include evaluation of ambulation tolerance, mobility restriction, inability to perform daily activities, and symptoms of altered mood and anxiety.

iii. Diagnostic Tests:

1. X-ray: Obtain standing radiographs, flexion, extension, and lateral bending to evaluate segmental instability and hardware migration.

2. CT scan: May reveal pseudarthrosis.

3. MRI: May be performed to evaluate for possible discogenic pathology or encroachment of the foramen. Utilization of contrast may be necessary if the patient has a history of discitis, osteomyelitis of the vertebral bodies, and/or differentiation of postoperative epidural fibrosis from recurrent disc herniation. MRI may reveal nerve root enhancement and/or thickening with extensive epidural fibrosis, which are related to recurrent or residual pathology.

4. Electrodiagnostic studies may be performed to differentiate from a peripheral neuropathy from a nerve root pathology.

TREATMENT

i. Medication therapy is directed toward the type of pain and the risk to benefit ratio of the pharmacotherapy. Medications may be used in combination with modalities such as thermotherapy and TENS units. Additionally, incorporation of physical therapy to develop a home therapeutic exercise program to increase spinal stability and prevent muscle atrophy.

ii. Procedural interventions include medial branch block, radiofrequency ablation, transforaminal epidural steroid injection, percutaneous epidural lysis of adhesions, and spinal cord stimulation.

1. Interlaminar epidural steroid injections are typically avoided because inability to obtain a perform the loss of resistance technique.

iii. Revision surgery may be considered in situations where there is evidence of hardware migration, segmental instability, or nerve root impingement.

SACROILIAC JOINT DYSFUNCTION

DEFINITION: An adult sacroiliac joint is C-shaped and is the largest axial and true diarthrodial joint surrounded by a fibrous capsule and functions as a triplanar shock absorber due to its complex multiaxial joint motion. Sacroiliac joint pain often arises from disruption of architecture or biomechanics of the sacroiliac joint.

RISK FACTORS

i. The most common cause of sacroiliitis is idiopathic and may occur acutely or gradually with cumulative trauma such as motor vehicle accidents, fall on buttock, inflammatory disease (i.e., ankylosing spondylitis, Crohn's disease, sarcoidosis), degenerative changes from osteoarthritis, and during pregnancy.

ii. The sacroiliac joint is also at risk of degeneration following lumbar spinal fusion surgery.

PATHOPHYSIOLOGY: The sacroiliac joint is a true synovial, diarthrodial joint. The sacroiliac joint ligaments and surrounding muscles (gluteus maximus, piriformis, bicep femoris, and psoas muscles) all affect the joint mobility and limit motion in all planes. The anterior sacroiliac joint is innervated by the ventral rami of L5 to S2. The posterior sacroiliac joint is innervated by the dorsal rami of the lateral branches of L4 to S3.

EPIDEMIOLOGY

i. Sacroiliac joint pain may be responsible for 10% to 26% of non-radicular low back pain based on the International Association of the Study of Pain criteria:

1. Pain in the sacroiliac joint region
2. SI joint provocation test reproduce the pain

ASSESSMENT:

i. History: Although there is no specific inciting event, for most patients, patients report pain over the sacroiliac joint primarily with sitting, and going up and down steps. Patients often report sacroiliac joint pain often mimicking sciatica.

ii. Physical Examination

1. Exam should begin with inspection to assess for any leg length discrepancy and asymmetry. A Fortin's sign may be present where there is tenderness to palpation within 1-cm inferior and medial to the posterior superior iliac spine.

2. Sacroiliac provocation tests: For a test to be positive, it must reproduce the patient's typical pain in the sacroiliac joint region. Three or more positive tests would increase sensitivity and specificity of SI joint as the pain generator.

   a. Distraction: Patient lies supine and is asked to place their forearms under their low back to maintain lumbar lordosis and to support the lumbar spine. Next, a pillow is placed under the patient's knees. The practitioner places their own hands on the anterior and medial aspect of the patient's left and right anterior superior iliac spine (ASIS) with arms crossed and elbow straight.

   b. Gaenslen's test: The patient is placed in a supine position with the affected side leg near the edge of the examination table. The unaffected extremity is kept in extension, whereas the tested leg is placed in maximal flexion. The practitioner places one hand on the anterior thigh of the nontested leg and the other hand on the knee of the tested leg to apply flexion. The extended leg may also be placed off the table to create a greater pressure.

   c. The practitioner flexes the nonsymptomatic hip, with the knee flexed up to 90 degrees. The patient should hold the asymptomatic leg with both arms while the practitioner stabilizes the pelvis and applies pressure to the sympathetic side and holds it in the hyperextended position while applying a downward force to the symptomatic side.

   d. Posterior shear (thigh thrust): With the patient lying supine and the affected side's hip flexed to approximately 90 degrees, the pelvis is stabilized at the opposite ASIS by the practitioner. The practitioner increases pressure through the axis of the femur.

   e. Patrick-FABER (Flexion, ABduction, External Rotation): While the patient is lying supine, the examiner crosses the patient's affected-side foot over the opposite-side thigh. The pelvis is stabilized at the opposite ASIS by the practitioner. Next, the practitioner applies a downward force to the affected-side's upper leg of the patient and is steadily increased, causing hip flexion, abduction, and external rotation.

f. Compression: The patient is asked to lie on the side with the affected side up and faced away from the practitioner. The practitioner then places a downward pressure through the anterior aspect of the lateral ilium, between the greater trochanter and iliac crest.

3. Gait evaluation should be performed for SI joint motion.

iii. Diagnostic Tests

1. Imaging

a. X-ray: AP sacrum x-ray, and modified Ferguson view on x-ray can help diagnose seronegative arthropatheis.

b. Bone scan may reveal infection, tumor, or arthritis.

c. MRI may reveal soft-tissue changes, infection, tumor, or arthritis.

d. Gold standard diagnostic test is a diagnostic and therapeutic sacroiliac joint injection.

TREATMENT

i. The treatment of sacroiliac joint dysfunction involves restoration of joint mechanics, improvement of trunk balance, and increasing lower extremity strength.

ii. A diagnostic and therapeutic sacroiliac joint injection

REHABILITATION PROGRAM

i. Modalities: Heat, ice, massage, electrical stimulation

ii. Stretching of iliotibial band, external hip rotators, hip flexors, and hamstrings

iii. Strengthening of core muscles and hip girdle

iv. Postural education

v. SI joints mobilization techniques

vi. Improvement of hip ROM

LUMBAR INTERLAMINAR EPIDURAL STEROID INJECTION

a. Indications: lumbar stenosis, lumbar radiculopathy, lumbar disc herniation

b. Contraindications:

   i. Absolute contraindications:

      1. Patient refusal

      2. Local or systemic injection

      3. Cauda equina syndrome

      4. Inadequate treatment of bleeding disorders which predispose to hemorrhage

      5. Allergy to medications or contrast used

   ii. Relative contraindications:

      1. Immunosuppressive state

      2. Pregnancy

      3. Inability to lie down (especially in conditions which may lead to respiratory distress)

      4. Untreated hypertension

      5. Untreated diabetes

      6. Concurrent use of anticoagulation or antiplatelet agents which may lead to bleeding and/or hematoma formation.

c. Functional anatomy:

   i. EPIDURAL SPACE BOUNDARIES

Anteriorly	Posterior longitudinal ligament, vertebral discs, and bodies
Posteriorly	Ligamentum flavum, capsule of facet joints, and laminae
Laterally	Pedicles and intervertebral foramina
Superiorly	Fusion of the spinal and periosteal layers of dura mater at the foramen magnum
Inferiorly	Sacrococcygeal membranes

ii. Order of encountered structures while performing a lumbar interlaminar epidural injection:

1. Skin
2. Subcutaneous tissue
3. Ligamentum nuchae or supraspinous ligament
4. Interspinous ligament
5. Ligamentum flavum
6. Epidural space

d. Recommended needle: 18- or 20-gauge, 3½ (or larger) Tuohy needle

e. Injectate: 3 mL to 4 mL normal saline, 12 mg betamethasone, or 10 mg dexamethasone

f. Contrast volume: 2 mL to 4 mL

g. Patient positioning: Place the patient in a prone position on the C-arm table.

h. C-Arm positions used: AP, lateral, and occasionally contralateral oblique

i. Technique:

i. Rotate the C-arm so the spinous processes are aligned midline in AP, and tilt the C-arm caudally so the end plates are aligned to show a single solid line rather than two individual lines.

ii. Prep the skin using a chlorhexidine prep (preferably), povidone iodine, isopropyl alcohol are all options for antiseptic agents for use in percutaneous spine procedures.

iii. Identify the appropriate interlaminar space with fluoroscopy using a radiopaque object such as a needle or metal marker to mark the space. Use a sterile marker if using a marker.

iv. Infiltrate the skin and subcutaneous tissues with 3 mL to 5 mL of 1% lidocaine using a 25- or 27-gauge needle. Inject into the deeper ligamentous structures for a better anesthetic effect.

v. With the C-arm in the AP position, the Tuohy needle is introduced midline approach with the tip of the needle directed toward the midline between spinous process of the level desired or to the ipsilateral side of the patient's pain.

vi. Advance the needle slowly with frequent confirmations of not crossing midline using the C-arm.

vii. The needle is advanced until the interspinous ligament is "subjectively" encountered.

viii. The C-arm is then rotated into a lateral position to allow confirmation of the depth.

ix. Now, based on the practitioner's preference, a loss of resistance (using air or saline) technique can be utilized to identify entrance into the epidural space. The needle stylet is removed and a syringe with either saline or air is attached to the hub of the needle.

x. The needle is stabilized by holding the wings and advanced slowly in the same trajectory and the "loss of resistance" is checked by gently tapping on the syringe plunger. Once the loss of resistance has occurred, the advancement of the needle should be stopped to prevent a "wet tap" or spinal cord injury. Needle advancement should be stopped if the patient develops severe pain or paresthesias. Make sure there is negative aspirate for air, cerebrospinal fluid (CSF), and blood.

xi. A negative aspiration check should be performed to ensure the needle is not placed into a blood vessel or CSF. Connect the extension tubing to the needle and under live fluoroscopy, confirmation of epidural space entrance is verified by injection of .5 mL to 2 mL of nonionic contrast to verify spread into the epidural space by obtaining both lateral and AP views.

xii. Digital subtraction can also be utilized to ensure absence of vascular flow.

xiii. After contrast confirmation of entry into the epidural space is done, the injectant mixture of corticosteroids and anesthetic is slowly injected.

xiv. The stylet is then reinserted into the needle, and the needle is withdrawn slowly.

xv. Place a gauze on the needle entry point and apply pressure if there is bleeding. Place the sterile dressing or bandage at the needle entry point.

xvi. Observe the patient postprocedure to assure that there are no adverse reactions. Provide the patient with postprocedure care instructions.

j. Complications:

i. Mild complications include self-limited bleeding which may induce postprocedure pain.

ii. Patient may also note myalgias or burning at the injection site several hours after the procedure due to the needle trauma.

iii. Postdural puncture ("wet tap") headache is another potential complication where the patient complains of headache that gets better after lying down. A blood patch may be indicated if the headache does not improve.

iv. Postprocedure hyperglycemia may also occur secondary to corticosteroids. Patients who are diabetic should be aware of this to determine if their diet and/or insulin regimen needs to be adjusted after the procedure.

v. More serious complications include the following:

   1. Epidural hematoma formation

   2. Arachnoiditis

   3. Intravascular injection—spinal cord ischemia

   4. Spinal cord injury

   5. Pneumothorax

k. Example: AP (Figure 6.2):

Figure 6.2: Anteroposterior view.

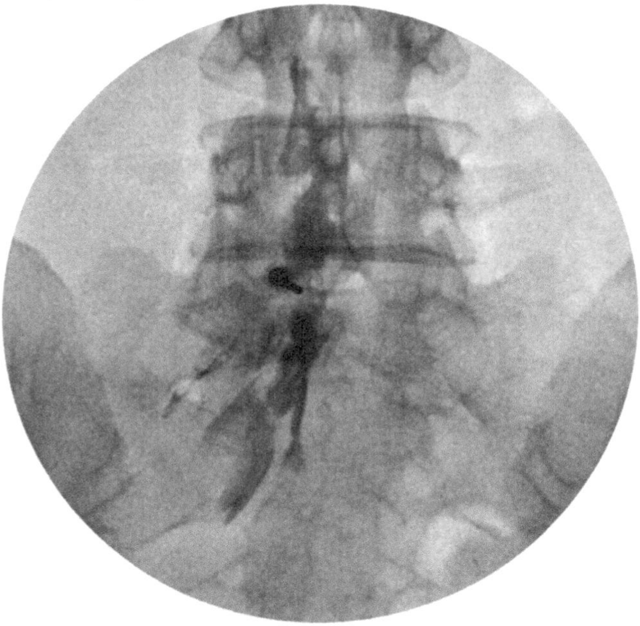

Sample Procedure Note

PREOPERATIVE DIAGNOSIS: Lumbar radiculitis
Lumbar spinal stenosis
Low back pain

POSTOPERATIVE DIAGNOSIS: Same
SURGEON: _____
ASSISTANT: _____
TITLE OF PROCEDURE: Lumbar epidural
steroid injection under
fluoroscopic guidance
Lumbar epidurogram

https://bcove.video/2jTfMgm   interpretation under
fluoroscopy (Video 6.1)

ANESTHESIA: Monitored anesthesia care
ESTIMATED BLOOD LOSS: None
COMPLICATIONS: None
DRAINS: None
IV Fluid 200 mL lactated ringer
IV, intravenous.

Indications: _____-year-old _____ (male/female) complaining of low back pain that radiates to the lower extremity. Our plan is to perform a lumbar epidural steroid injection under fluoroscopic guidance today. The risks and benefits of _____ lumbar epidural steroid injection were discussed in detail. The patient understands and accepts that the risks include, but are not limited to, increase in pain, nerve injury, infection, bleeding, hematoma, paralysis, spinal headache, stroke, discitis, and death. Alternatives to nerve blocks, or noninterventional therapy, were discussed and informed consent obtained.

DESCRIPTION OF PROCEDURE

Intravenous access was established. The patient was escorted to the fluoroscopy suite and placed in the prone position. Noninvasive monitoring was applied. Universal Site and Side Protocol was followed and documented. Safe Injection and Infection Control Practices as recommended by the Center for

(continued)

(continued)

Disease Control, including the use of a face mask, were strictly followed. The lumbar area is widely prepped using isopropyl alcohol per protocol, and sterile drapes applied. Time-out was performed. Using fluoroscopic guidance, the lumbar vertebral bodies were identified. Using a 25-gauge needle, a skin wheal was raised with 1% lidocaine. Under fluoroscopic guidance in the AP and lateral views, an 18-gauge modified winged Tuohy needle was placed at the _____ interspace. The Tuohy needle was carried down to the epidural space using intermittent loss of resistance technique with air to identify the epidural space. Once the epidural space was identified AP and lateral projections of the fluoroscope confirmed adequate needle placement. At this point, 2 mL of Omnipaque-240 contrast was injected under live fluoroscopic guidance outlining a positive epidurogram. There was no evidence of intrathecal or intravascular spread. After negative aspiration for heme and CSF, 40 mg of Kenalog with _____mL of .25% preservative-free bupivacaine was injected without complication. Once the procedure was completed, all needles were withdrawn from the patient intact. A bandage was applied to the puncture site. The patient tolerated this procedure well, there were no complications noted. The patient was discharged in hemodynamically and neurologically stable condition, with review of postprocedural instructions.

Plan: If the patient received 50% or greater improvement of their pain, we will repeat the procedure in 2 to 4 weeks' time. If today's injection does not alleviate the patient's pain by 50%, we will perform a diagnostic lumbar transforaminal epidural steroid injection fluoroscopic guidance in 2 to 3 weeks.

_____

Attending Physician

LUMBAR TRANSFORAMINAL EPIDURAL STEROID INJECTIONS

a. Indications: lumbar radiculopathy, lumbar neuroforaminal stenosis, lumbar stenosis, lumbar herniated disks

b. Contraindications:

    i. Absolute contraindications:

        1. Patient refusal

        2. Local or systemic injection

        3. Cauda equina syndrome

        4. Inadequate treatment of bleeding disorders which predispose to hemorrhage

        5. Allergy to medications or contrast used

    ii. Relative contraindications:

        1. Immunosuppressive state

        2. Pregnancy

        3. Inability to lie down (especially in conditions which may lead to respiratory distress)

        4. Untreated hypertension

        5. Untreated diabetes

        6. Concurrent use of anticoagulation or antiplatelet agents, which may lead to bleeding and/or hematoma formation.

c. Recommended needle: 22- or 25-gauge, 3½ (or longer) Quincke spinal needle

d. Injectate: 2 mL to 3 mL of 0.9% normal saline (or .25% bupivacaine) and 12 mg of betamethasone (or 8–10 mg of dexamethasone)

e. Contrast volume: 2 mL to 4 mL

f. Patient positioning: Place the patient in a prone position on the C-arm table.

g. C-arm positioning: Ipsilateral oblique, lateral, AP

h. Technique:

    i. Prep the skin using a chlorhexidine prep (preferably), povidone iodine, isopropyl alcohol are all options for antiseptic agents for use in percutaneous spine procedures.

ii. Under AP view, identify the correct lumbar level with fluoroscopy using a radiopaque object such as needle or metal marker to identify the correct level.

iii. Tilt the fluoroscope with caudad or cephalad to align the superior endplates.

iv. Oblique the C-arm ipsilaterally until the targeted neural foramen is visualized.

v. Infiltrate the skin and subcutaneous tissues with 3 mL to 5 mL of 1% lidocaine using a 25- or 27-gauge needle. Inject into the deeper ligamentous structures for a better anesthetic effect.

vi. Advance the needle using intermittent fluoroscopy toward the superior, lateral, and anterior aspect of the neural foramen. This area is often referred to as the safe triangle (Figure 6.3).

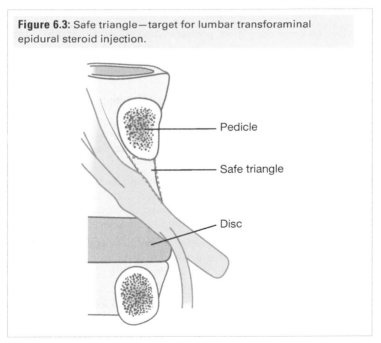

Figure 6.3: Safe triangle—target for lumbar transforaminal epidural steroid injection.

Pedicle

Safe triangle

Disc

vii. Obtain AP view on the C-arm to ensure the needle is advanced toward the 6 o'clock position of the pedicle.

    viii. Next, under lateral view, advance the needle to the spinol-aminar line.

    ix. Return back to the AP view and connect the extension tubing to the needle.

    x. After negative aspiration, inject nonionic contrast to verify outline of the targeted nerve root.

    xi. Digital subtraction can also be utilized to ensure absence of vascular flow.

    xii. After contrast confirmation, the injectant mixture of corticosteroids and anesthetic is slowly injected.

    xiii. The stylet is then reinserted into the needle, and the needle is withdrawn slowly.

    xiv. Place a gauze on the needle entry point and apply pressure if there is bleeding. Place the sterile dressing or bandage at the needle entry point.

    xv. Observe the patient postprocedure to assure that there are no adverse reactions. Provide the patient with postprocedure care instructions.

i. Complications:

    i. Mild complications include self-limited bleeding which may induce postprocedure pain.

    ii. Patient may also note myalgias or burning at the injection site several hours after the procedure due to the needle trauma.

    iii. Postdural puncture ("wet tap") headache is another potential complication where the patient complains of headache that gets better after lying down. A blood patch may be indicated if the headache does not improve.

    iv. Postprocedure hyperglycemia may also occur secondary to corticosteroids. Patients who are diabetic should be aware of this to see if their diet and/or insulin regimen needs to be adjusted after the procedure.

    v. More serious complications include the following:

        1. Epidural hematoma formation

        2. Arachnoiditis

        3. Intravascular injection—spinal cord ischemia

        4. Spinal cord injury

        5. Pneumothorax

j. Examples: AP (Figures 6.4 and 6.6) and lateral (Figure 6.5):

Figure 6.4: Epidural spread with an S1 transforaminal epidural steroid injection with S1 nerve root outlined by contrast.

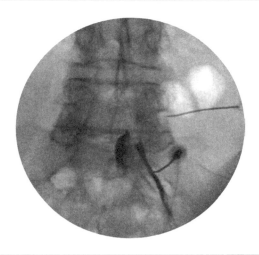

Figure 6.5: Lateral view while performing an L5 and S1 transforaminal epidural steroid injection.

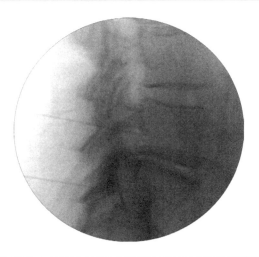

Figure 6.6: Contrast outlining an L5 and S1 lumbar transforaminal epidural steroid injection.

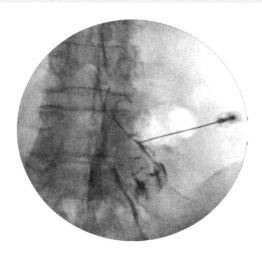

Sample Procedure Note

PREOPERATIVE DIAGNOSIS:	Lumbar radiculitis Lumbar disc displacement Low back pain
POSTOPERATIVE DIAGNOSIS:	Same
SURGEON:	_____
ASSISTANT:	_____
TITLE OF PROCEDURE:	Diagnostic _____ lumbar transforaminal epidural steroid injection under fluoroscopic guidance with lumbar epidurogram interpretation under fluoroscopy (**Videos 6.2 and 6.3**)
ANESTHESIA:	Monitored anesthesia care
ESTIMATED BLOOD LOSS:	None

https://bcove.video/2Ij4UqP

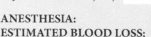

https://bcove.video/2Ij5HIj

(continued)

(continued)

COMPLICATIONS:	None
DRAINS:	None
IV Fluid	200 mL lactated ringer
IV, intravenous.	

Indications: _____-year-old _____ (male/female) complaining of low back pain that radiates to the lower extremity. Our plan is to perform a lumbar transforaminal epidural steroid injection under fluoroscopic guidance today. The risks and benefits of _____ a lumbar transforaminal epidural steroid injection were discussed in detail. The patient understands and accepts that the risks include, but are not limited to, increase in pain, nerve injury, infection, bleeding, hematoma, paralysis, spinal headache, stroke, discitis, and death. Alternatives to nerve blocks, or noninterventional therapy, were discussed and informed consent obtained.

DESCRIPTION OF PROCEDURE
Intravenous access was established. The patient was escorted to the fluoroscopy suite and placed in the prone position. Noninvasive monitoring was applied. Universal Site and Side Protocol was followed and documented. Safe Injection and Infection Control Practices as recommended by the Center for Disease Control, including the use of a face mask, were strictly followed. The lumbar area is widely prepped using isopropyl alcohol per protocol, and sterile drapes applied. Time-out was performed. Using fluoroscopic guidance, the lumbar vertebral bodies were identified. Using a 25-gauge needle, a skin wheal was raised with 1% lidocaine. The fluoroscope was obliqued 20 degrees to the _____ with a cephalocaudal tilt to align the vertebral endplates and outline the landmark of the Scotty dog. A 22-gauge 5-inch curved Quincke spinal needle was placed at the 6 o'clock position of the Scotty dog at the _____ vertebral body. Each needle was independently carried down to the neural foramen under fluoroscopic guidance. Once the neural foramen was entered, AP and lateral projections of the fluoroscope confirmed adequate needle placement. At this time, 2 mL of Omnipaque-240 contrast was injected under live fluoroscopic guidance through a T-Connector extension tubing outlining a positive neurogram and an epidurogram. There was no evidence of intrathecal or

(*continued*)

> intravascular spread. After negative aspiration for heme and CSF, _____mg of _____ with 1 mL of .25% preservative-free bupivacaine was injected without complication. Once the procedure was completed, all needles were withdrawn from the patient intact. A bandage was applied to the puncture site. The patient tolerated this procedure well, there were no complications noted. The patient was discharged in hemodynamically and neurologically stable condition, with review of postprocedural instructions.
>
> **Plan:** If the patient received 50% or greater improvement of their pain, we will repeat the procedure in 2 to 4 weeks' time. If today's injection does not alleviate the patient's pain by 50%, we will perform a diagnostic lumbar medial branch block under fluoroscopic guidance in 2 to 3 weeks.
>
> _____
> **Attending Physician**

CAUDAL EPIDURAL STEROID INJECTION

a. Indications: lumbar radiculopathy, lumbar stenosis, lumbar herniated disks, history of lumbar laminectomy, or fusion
b. Contraindications:
   i. Absolute contraindications:
      1. Patient refusal
      2. Local or systemic injection
      3. Cauda equina syndrome
      4. Inadequate treatment of bleeding disorders which predispose to hemorrhage
      5. Allergy to medications or contrast used
   ii. Relative contraindications:
      1. Immunosuppressive state
      2. Pregnancy

   3. Inability to lie down (especially in conditions which may lead to respiratory distress)

   4. Untreated hypertension

   5. Untreated diabetes

   6. Concurrent use of anticoagulation or antiplatelet agents which may lead to bleeding and/or hematoma formation.

c. Recommended needle: 22- or 25-gauge, 3½ (or longer) Quincke spinal needle

d. Injectate: 4 mL to 5 mL of 0.9% normal saline, 3 mL of 1% lidocaine (or .25% bupivacaine) and 12 mg of betamethasone (or 80 mg of triamcinolone)

e. Contrast volume: 2 mL to 4 mL

f. Patient positioning: Place the patient in a prone position on the C-arm table.

g. C-arm positioning: Lateral and AP

h. Technique:

   i. Prep the skin using a chlorhexidine prep (preferably), povidone iodine, isopropyl alcohol are all options for antiseptic agents for use in percutaneous spine procedures.

   ii. Rotate the C-arm in the lateral position.

   iii. Palpate and then identify the sacral hiatus under lateral fluoroscopy.

   iv. Infiltrate the skin and subcutaneous tissues with 3 mL to 5 mL of 1% lidocaine using a 25- or 27-gauge needle. Inject into the deeper ligamentous structures for a better anesthetic effect.

   v. Insert the Quincke spinal needle over the anesthetized skin at a 30 degree angle to the sacrum.

   vi. Advance the needle tip through the sacral hiatus and continue driving the needle parallel to the sacrum to below the S2 segment.

   vii. A negative aspiration check should be performed to ensure the needle is not placed into a blood vessel or CSF. Connect the extension tubing to the needle and under live fluoroscopy, confirmation of epidural space entrance is verified by injection of 0.5 mL to 2 mL of nonionic contrast to verify spread into the epidural space by obtaining both lateral and AP views.

   viii. Digital subtraction can also be utilized to ensure absence of vascular flow.

    ix. After contrast confirmation of entry into the epidural space is done, the injectant mixture of corticosteroids and anesthetic is slowly injected.

     x. The stylet is then reinserted into the needle, and the needle is withdrawn slowly.

    xi. Place a gauze on the needle entry point and apply pressure if there is bleeding. Place the sterile dressing or bandage at the needle entry point.

    xii. Observe the patient postprocedure to assure that there are no adverse reactions. Provide the patient with postprocedure care instructions.

i. Complications

    i. Mild complications include self-limited bleeding which may induce postprocedure pain.

   ii. Patient may also note myalgias or burning at the injection site several hours after the procedure due to the needle trauma.

  iii. Postdural puncture ("wet tap") headache is another potential complication where the patient complains of headache that gets better after lying down. A blood patch may be indicated if the headache does not improve.

  iv. Postprocedure hyperglycemia may also occur secondary to corticosteroids. Patients who are diabetic should be aware of this to determine if their diet and/or insulin regimen needs to be adjusted after the procedure.

   v. More serious complications include the following:

    1. Due to a large volume injectate, cauda equina syndrome may occur due to reduction of the epidural space.

    2. Epidural hematoma formation

    3. Arachnoiditis

    4. Intravascular injection—spinal cord ischemia

    5. Spinal cord injury

    6. Pneumothorax

    7. Worsening of epidural lipomatosis

j. Examples (Figures 6.7 and 6.8):

Figure 6.7: Lateral view of the needle traversing past the sacrococcygeal ligament and membrane.

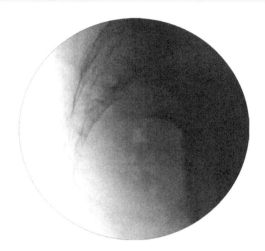

Figure 6.8: Anterior posterior view of the epidural contrast spread with highlighting the right S1 nerve root.

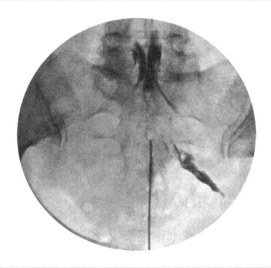

Sample Procedure Note

PREOPERATIVE DIAGNOSIS:	Lumbar radiculitis
	Lumbar disc displacement
	Low back pain
POSTOPERATIVE DIAGNOSIS:	Same
SURGEON:	_____
ASSISTANT:	_____
TITLE OF PROCEDURE:	Caudal epidural
	steroid injection under
	fluoroscopic guidance
	Lumbar epidurogram
	interpretation under
	fluoroscopy (**Video 6.4**)
ANESTHESIA:	Monitored anesthesia care
ESTIMATED BLOOD LOSS:	None
COMPLICATIONS:	None
DRAINS:	None
IV Fluid	200 mL lactated ringer

 https://bcove.video/2rGPbYt

IV, intravenous.

Indications: _____ year-old _____ (male/female) complaining of low back pain that radiates to the lower extremity. Our plan is to perform a caudal epidural steroid injection under fluoroscopic guidance today. The risks and benefits of a caudal epidural steroid injection were discussed in detail. The patient understands and accepts that the risks include but are not limited to, increase in pain, nerve injury, infection, bleeding, hematoma, paralysis, spinal headache, stroke, discitis, and death. Alternatives to nerve blocks, or noninterventional therapy, were discussed and informed consent obtained.

DESCRIPTION OF PROCEDURE
Intravenous access was established. The patient was escorted to the fluoroscopy suite and placed in the prone position. Noninvasive monitoring was applied. Universal Site and Side Protocol was followed and documented. Safe Injection and Infection Control Practices as recommended by the Center for Disease Control, including the use of a face mask, were

(continued)

(continued)

strictly followed. The lumbo sacral area and buttock is widely prepped using isopropyl alcohol per protocol, and sterile drapes applied. Time-out was performed. Using fluoroscopic guidance the caudal canal was easily identified. Using a 25-gauge needle, a skin wheal was raised with 1% lidocaine. Under fluoroscopic guidance in the AP and lateral views, an 18-gauge modified winged Tuohy needle was placed into the caudal canal without difficulty. Once the caudal canal was entered, AP and lateral projections of the fluoroscope confirmed adequate needle placement. At this point, 2 mL of Omnipaque-240 contrast was injected under live fluoroscopic guidance outlining a positive epidurogram. There was no evidence of intrathecal or intravascular spread. After negative aspiration for heme and CSF, 40 mg of triamcinolone with _____mL of 0.25% preservative-free bupivacaine was injected without complication. Once the procedure was completed, all needles were withdrawn from the patient intact. A bandage was applied to the puncture site. The patient tolerated this procedure well, there were no complications noted. The patient was discharged in hemodynamically and neurologically stable condition, with review of postprocedural instructions.

Plan: If the patient received 50% or greater improvement of their pain, we will repeat the procedure in 2 to 4 weeks' time. If today's injection does not alleviate the patient's pain by 50%, we will perform a diagnostic lumbar transforaminal epidural steroid injection fluoroscopic guidance in 2 to 3 weeks.

Attending Physician

LUMBAR MEDIAL BRANCH BLOCK

a. Indications: Lumbar facet arthropathy, lumbar spondylosis, lumbar spondylolysis
b. Contraindications:

    i. Absolute contraindications:

       1. Patient refusal

       2. Local or systemic injection

       3. Cauda equina syndrome

       4. Inadequate treatment of bleeding disorders which predispose to hemorrhage

       5. Allergy to medications or contrast used

    ii. Relative contraindications:

       1. Immunosuppressive state

       2. Pregnancy

       3. Inability to lie down (especially in conditions which may lead to respiratory distress)

       4. Untreated hypertension

       5. Untreated diabetes

       6. Concurrent use of anticoagulation or antiplatelet agents which may lead to bleeding and/or hematoma formation

c. Recommended needle: 22- or 25-gauge, 3½-inch (or longer) Quincke spinal needle

d. Injectate: .5 mL of 1% lidocaine (or .25%–.75% of bupivacaine) per medial branch block

e. Contrast volume: up to .5 mL

f. C-arm positioning: AP, ipsilateral oblique, and lateral views

g. Technique:

    i. Prep the skin using a chlorhexidine prep (preferably), povidone iodine, isopropyl alcohol are all options for antiseptic agents for use in percutaneous spine procedures.

    ii. Identify the target levels using AP view on the C-arm.

    iii. Tilt the fluoroscopy caudad or cephalad to align the endplates.

    iv. Next, ipsilaterally oblique the C-arm to visualize the "eye" of the Scotty dog—also known as the pedicle. The target point for the L1L4 medial branches is the 11 o'clock position on the left-sided pedicles or the 2 o'clock position on the right-sided pedicles. This area is the junction of the superior articular process and the transverse process, where the medial branches lie. If targeting the L5S1 facet joint, the target is the sacral ala where the L5 dorsal ramus is located, also known as the junction of the sacral ala and the base of the S1 superior articular process.

  v. Infiltrate the skin and subcutaneous tissues with 3 mL to 5 mL of 1% lidocaine using a 25- or 27-gauge needle. Direct the needle in the same projected trajectory of the medial branch block. Inject into the deeper ligamentous structures for a better anesthetic effect.

 vi. After identification of the levels to be blocked, a 22- or 25-gauge, 2- to 3-inch spinal needle can be inserted through the skin.

vii. Advance the spinal needle with intermittent fluoroscopy checks. Once the needle reaches the bone, it can be retracted slightly and the trajectory can be placed laterally to the deepest concave point, the location of the medial branches. The needle point should be at the lateral margin of the articular process.

viii. After a negative aspiration, inject anesthetic mixture. Contrast may also be used for further confirmation.

 ix. The patient should be instructed to assess his or her pain relief in 30 minute to 1 hour increments immediately following the diagnostic blocks. The patient should also be instructed to not modify their activity postprocedure to ensure authentic results. A positive diagnostic block should demonstrate at least 50% reduction in pain. If successful, the procedure should be repeated at least one additional time to verify reproducibility before proceeding with a radiofrequency procedure.

  x. Complications:

   1. Transient neuritis and/or burning sensation in the treated spinal nerve

   2. Dural puncture

   3. Spinal cord trauma

   4. Spinal anesthesia

   5. Meningitis, neural trauma

   6. Pneumothorax

   7. Facet capsule rupture

   8. Hematoma formation

Sample Procedure Note

PREOPERATIVE DIAGNOSIS: Lumbar spondylosis
Lumbar disc displacement
Low back pain

POSTOPERATIVE DIAGNOSIS: Same
SURGEON: _____
ASSISTANT: _____
TITLE OF PROCEDURE: Diagnostic _____
lumbar medial branch
block under fluoroscopic
guidance (**Videos 6.5, 6.6, and 6.7**)

 https://bcove.video/2IkZEik

 https://bcove.video/2Kip1Ss

https://bcove.video/2IeGX3X

ANESTHESIA: Monitored anesthesia care
ESTIMATED BLOOD LOSS: None
COMPLICATIONS: None
DRAINS: None
IV Fluid 200 mL lactated ringer
IV, intravenous.

Indications: _____-year-old _____ (male/female) complaining of low back pain with reproducible facet tenderness to palpation. The pain does not radiate to the lower extremity. Our plan is to perform a diagnostic lumbar medial branch block under fluoroscopic guidance today. The risks and benefits of _____ median branch nerve blocks were discussed in detail. The patient understands and accepts that the risks include, but are not limited to, increase in pain, nerve injury, infection, bleeding, hematoma, paralysis, spinal headache, stroke, discitis, and death. Alternatives to nerve blocks, or noninterventional therapy, were discussed and informed consent obtained.

(continued)

(continued)

DESCRIPTION OF PROCEDURE
Intravenous access was established. The patient was escorted
to the fluoroscopy suite and placed in the prone position.
Noninvasive monitoring was applied. Universal Site and Side
Protocol was followed and documented. Safe Injection and
Infection Control Practices as recommended by the Center
for Disease Control, including the use of a face mask, were
strictly followed. The lumbar area is widely prepped using
isopropyl alcohol per protocol, and sterile drapes applied.
Time-out was performed. The fluoroscope was obliqued 20
degrees to the _____ with a cephalocaudad tilt to identify
the landmark of the Scotty dog. Using a 25-gauge needle, a
skin wheal was raised with 1% lidocaine. Under fluoroscopic
guidance, a 22-gauge 3.5-inch curved Quincke spinal needle
was advanced into the eye of the pedicle of the _____
vertebral body. AP and lateral projections of the fluoroscope
confirmed adequate needle placement. Needle placement was
then confirmed using .2 mL of Omnipaque-240 contrast at
each level. There was no evidence of intrathecal, epidural, or
intravascular spread. After negative aspiration for heme and
CSF, a total volume of .5 mL of .75% bupivacaine was injected
through the needle at each level to block the corresponding
medial branch nerve. Once the procedure was completed, all
needles were withdrawn from the patient intact. A bandage
was applied to the puncture site. The patient tolerated this
sequence well, there were no complications noted. The patient
was discharged in hemodynamically and neurologically stable
condition, with review of postprocedural instructions. The
patient was given a pain diary with usage instructions. We
will review the patients' pain diary in consideration for a
possible corresponding lumbar medial branch radiofrequency
thermal coagulation.

_____

Attending Physician

h. Examples (Figures 6.9, 6.10, and 6.11):

Figure 6.9: Anterior posterior view of the lumbar medial branch block with contrast.

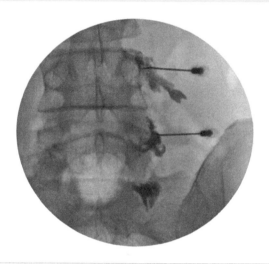

Figure 6.10: Lateral view of the lumbar medial branch block.

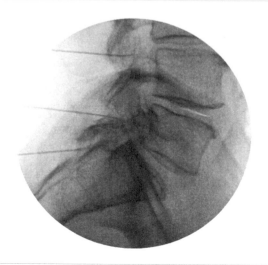

Figure 6.11: Intra-articular facet joint injection.

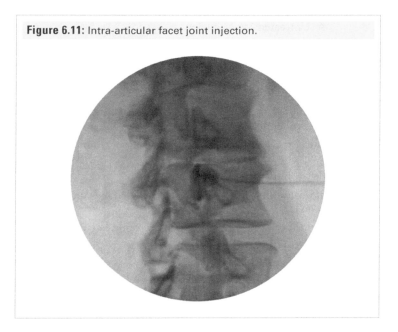

SACROILIAC JOINT INJECTION

a. Indications: Sacroiliac joint pain, sacrococcygeal ligament pain
b. Contraindications:
    i. Absolute contraindications:
        1. Patient refusal
        2. Local or systemic injection
        3. Cauda equina syndrome
        4. Inadequate treatment of bleeding disorders which predispose to hemorrhage
        5. Allergy to medications or contrast used.
    ii. Relative contraindications:
        1. Immunosuppressive state
        2. Pregnancy
        3. Inability to lie down (especially in conditions which may lead to respiratory distress)

4. Untreated hypertension

5. Untreated diabetes

6. Concurrent use of anticoagulation or antiplatelet agents which may lead to bleeding and/or hematoma formation.

c. Recommended needle: 22- or 25-gauge, 3½-inch (or longer) Quincke spinal needle

d. Injectate: 1 mL of 1% lidocaine and 40 mg of triamcinolone or 12 mg of betamethasone

e. Contrast volume: .25 mL to .50 mL

f. Patient positioning: Place the patient in a prone position on the C-arm table.

g. C-arm positioning: Contralateral oblique and lateral

h. Technique:

i. Prep the skin using a chlorhexidine prep (preferably), povidone iodine, isopropyl alcohol are all options for antiseptic agents for use in percutaneous spine procedures.

ii. Rotate the C-arm in the contralateral oblique to visualize the superimposed anterior and posterior surfaces of the sacroiliac joint.

iii. Anesthetize the skin over the needle entry site using a 25-gauge needle with 1% lidocaine.

iv. Insert and advance the spinal needle through the anesthetized skin to the target zone (lower one third of the visualized joint space). A "pop" may be felt once passing through the sacroiliac ligament.

v. Remove the stylet and connect an extension tubing to the needle and inject contrast dye with live fluoroscopy to assure that there is no intravascular spread.

vi. Once an arthrogram is achieved, inject the steroid mixture.

vii. The stylet is then reinserted into the needle, and the needle is withdrawn slowly.

viii. Place a gauze on the needle entry point and apply pressure if there is bleeding. Place the sterile dressing or bandage at the needle entry point.

ix. Observe the patient postprocedure to assure that there are no adverse reactions. Provide the patient with postprocedure care instructions.

Sample Procedure Note

PREOPERATIVE DIAGNOSIS:	Sacroiliitis
	Low back pain
POSTOPERATIVE DIAGNOSIS:	Same
SURGEON:	_____
ASSISTANT:	_____
TITLE OF PROCEDURE:	_____ Sacroiliac joint injection under fluoroscopic guidance (Video 6.8)

https://bcove.video/2IkzJHJ

ANESTHESIA:	Monitored anesthesia care
ESTIMATED BLOOD LOSS:	None
COMPLICATIONS:	None
DRAINS:	None
IV Fluid	200 mL lactated ringer

IV, intravenous.

Indications: _____-year-old _____ (male/female) complaining of pain over the sacroiliac joint. Our plan is to perform a sacroiliac joint injection under fluoroscopic guidance today. The risks and benefits of _____ sacroiliac joint injection were discussed in detail. The patient understands and accepts that the risks include, but are not limited to, increase in pain, nerve injury, infection, bleeding, hematoma, paralysis, spinal headache, stroke, discitis, and death. Alternatives to nerve blocks, or noninterventional therapy, were discussed and informed consent obtained.

DESCRIPTION OF PROCEDURE
Intravenous access was established. The patient was escorted to the fluoroscopy suite and placed in the prone position. Noninvasive monitoring was applied. Universal Site and Side Protocol was followed and documented. Safe Injection and Infection Control Practices as recommended by the Center for Disease Control, including the use of a face mask, were strictly followed. The sacroiliac joint and low back area is widely prepped using isopropyl alcohol per protocol, and sterile drapes applied. Time-out was performed. With the fluoroscope oblique 20 degrees the sacroiliac joint was easily identified. Using a 25-gauge needle,

(continued)

(continued)

a skin wheal was raised with 1% lidocaine. Under fluoroscopic guidance in the oblique and lateral views, a 22-gauge 3.5-inch curved spinal needle was placed into the SI joint on the _____. At this point, 2 mL Omnipaque-240 contrast was injected under live fluoroscopic guidance outlining a positive arthrogram. There was no evidence of intrathecal or intravascular spread. After negative aspiration for heme and CSF, 40 mg of Kenalog was injected with _____ mL of preservative-free _____ marcaine without complication. Once the procedure was completed, all needles were withdrawn from the patient intact. A bandage was applied to the puncture site. The patient tolerated this procedure well, there were no complications noted. The patient was discharged in hemodynamically and neurologically stable condition, with review of postprocedural instructions.

Plan: If the patient received 50% or greater improvement of their pain, we will repeat the procedure in 2 to 4 weeks' time. If today's injection does not alleviate the patient's pain by 50%, we will perform a diagnostic lumbar medial branch block under fluoroscopic guidance in 2 to 3 weeks.

_____

Attending Physician

i. Examples (Figures 6.12, 6.13, and 6.14):

Figure 6.12: Anterior posterior view of an intra-articular sacroiliac joint injection.

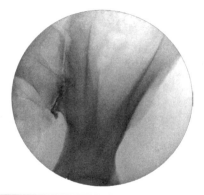

Figure 6.13: Anterior posterior view of an intra-articular sacroiliac joint injection with contrast highlight anterior and posterior portion of the joint.

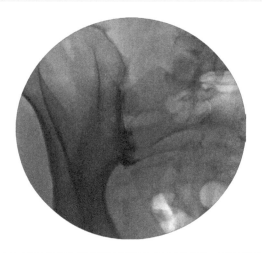

Figure 6.14: Anterior posterior view of an intra-articular sacroiliac joint injection.

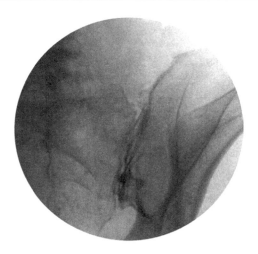

PROCEDURES AND ASSOCIATED CPT CODES

PROCEDURES	
Lumbar interlaminar epidural or caudal epidural steroid injection	**62323**
Lumbar transforaminal first level	**64483**
Lumbar transforaminal additional level	**64484**
Lumbar medial branch block or intra-articular facet joint injection first level	**64493**
Lumbar medial branch block or intra-articular facet joint injection second level	**64494**
Lumbar medial branch block or intra-articular facet joint injection third level	**64495**
Bilateral modifier	**50**
RFA—first lumbar level	**64635**
RFA additional levels	**64636**
Sacroiliac joint injection with fluoroscopy	**27096**
Sacroiliac joint RFA	
RF of L5 dorsal ramus	**64635**
RF of S1 lateral branches	**64640**
RF of S2 lateral branches	**64640**
RF of S3 lateral branch	**64640**
INJECTABLES	**J-codes**
Low osmolar contrast material (Omnipaque 300)	**Q9967**
Low osmolar contrast material (Omnipaque 240)	**Q9966**
Betamethasone (Celestone 3 mg)	**J0702**
Betamethasone (Celestone 4 mg)	**J0704**
Dexamethasone sodium phosphate 1 mg	**J1100**
Depo-Medrol (40 mg)	**J1030**
Depo-Medrol (80 mg)	**J1040**

(continued)

(*continued*)

Triamcinolone (per 10 mg)	**J3301**
Diphenhydramine (injection up to 50 mg)	**J1200**
Versed (per milligram)	**J2250**
Fentanyl (0.1 mg)	**J3010**

RF, radiofrequency; RFA, radiofrequency ablation.

List of Videos

 Video 6.1 Lumbar Interlaminar Epidural Steroid Injection

https://bcove.video/2jTfMgm

Video 6.2 Lumbar Transforaminal Epidural Steroid Injection

https://bcove.video/2Ij4UqP

 Video 6.3 S1 Transforaminal Epidural Steroid Injection

https://bcove.video/2Ij5HIj

Video 6.4 Caudal Epidural Steroid Injection

https://bcove.video/2rGPbYt

 Video 6.5 Thoracolumbar Radiofrequency Thermocoagulation

https://bcove.video/2IkZEik

Video 6.6 Lumbar Facet Injection

https://bcove.video/2Kip1Ss

Video 6.7 Lumbar Radiofrequency Ablation

https://bcove.video/2IeGX3X

Video 6.8 Sacroiliac Joint Injection

https://bcove.video/2IkzJHJ

Sympathetic Blocks

STELLATE GANGLION BLOCK

ANATOMY: The sympathetic chain lies in the fascial plane along the anterolateral portion of the vertebral bodies. In the majority of individuals, the first thoracic and inferior cervical ganglia are fused together to form what is called the "stellate ganglion." The stellate ganglion sits anterior to the neck of the first rib and the C7 transverse process and is anteromedial to the vertebral artery. The stellate ganglion is posterior to the common carotid artery, dome of the pleura, phrenic nerve, and the internal jugular vein. Medially, its borders include the vertebral column, esophagus, and trachea.

INDICATIONS: Pain syndromes involving the upper extremities and face:

- Complex regional pain syndrome (CRPS) I and II
- Neuropathic pain syndromes (shingles, postradiation neuritis, etc.)
- Lymphedema
- Phantom limb pain syndrome
- Cancer pain
- Differentiation of sympathetically mediated pain versus sympathetic independent pain of the head or upper extremity
- Head and face sympathetically mediated cancer pain
- Postmastectomy pain syndrome

CONTRAINDICATIONS

- Cardiac conduction block
- Risk of bullous puncture in patient with bullous emphysema
- Systemic or local infection in the area of the injection
- Coagulopathy
- Anterior lower cervical surgery

- Patient refusal
- Myocardial infarction (MI) within 12 weeks

TECHNIQUE

- Patient position: Supine and head neutral or slightly rotated to contralateral side of the procedure. A small shoulder roll may help align the cervical spine and chest.
- Recommended needle: 22- or 25-gauge, 3½-inch Quincke spinal needle
- Injectate: test dose of .5 mL to 1 mL of 1% lidocaine; once confirmed 10 mL of anesthetic is injected
- Contrast volume: 1 mL to 2 mL (Figure 7.1)
- C-arm position: anteroposterior (AP) view with a caudal tilt of the image intensifier to visualize the C6C7 disc space
- Medication: .25% bupivacaine or 1% lidocaine; triamcinolone or methylprednisolone (optional)
- Technique:
  1. Prep the skin in sterile fashion.
  2. Identify C6 or C7 transverse process on the fluoroscope.
  3. Usually performed at C6 between the trachea and carotid, at the level of the cricoid. The target is to make contact with the C6 bony prominence (also known as Chassaignac's tubercle).
  4. Using a 22-gauge 4- or 5-cm needle, the needle is advanced downward and perpendicular to the table plane toward the C6 transverse process. Once the needle is in direct contact with the C6 transverse process, the needle is withdrawn approximately 1 mm to 2 mm and contrast is injected which should spread cephalad and caudad between the tissue planes.
  5. Pooling of contrast indicates that the needle is in the longus colli muscle (Figures 7.1 and 7.2).
  6. Immediate disappearance of contrast indicates needle is intravascular, intrathecal, or intrapleural.
  7. 10 mL to 15 mL of anesthetic with intermittent aspiration is then injected.
  8. Successful blockade is typically achieved if the patient develops Horner's syndrome (ptosis, miosis, and anhydrosis).
  9. The patient should be monitored and observed for approximately 30 minutes following the procedure.

COMPLICATIONS

- Blocking at C7 (normal anatomical location) has a higher risk of causing a pneumothorax when compared to the C6 level and contrast injected at C6 level reached the C7T1 level consistently.
- Hoarseness if recurrent laryngeal nerve is blocked
- Hemidiaphragm if the phrenic nerve is blocked
- Carotid hematoma
- Internal jugular vein trauma
- Brachial plexus injury
- Hemothorax
- Chylothorax if the thoracic duct is injured
- Esophageal perforation
- Seizure if local anesthetic is injected intravascular
- Spinal cord injury
- Retropharyngeal hematoma

EXAMPLES

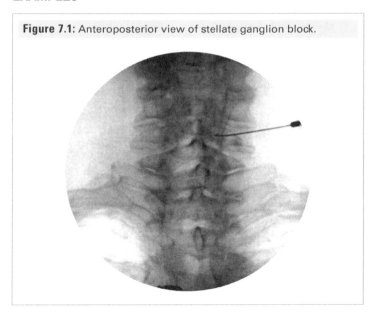

Figure 7.1: Anteroposterior view of stellate ganglion block.

Figure 7.2: Anteroposterior view of stellate ganglion block with contrast spread both cephalad and caudad.

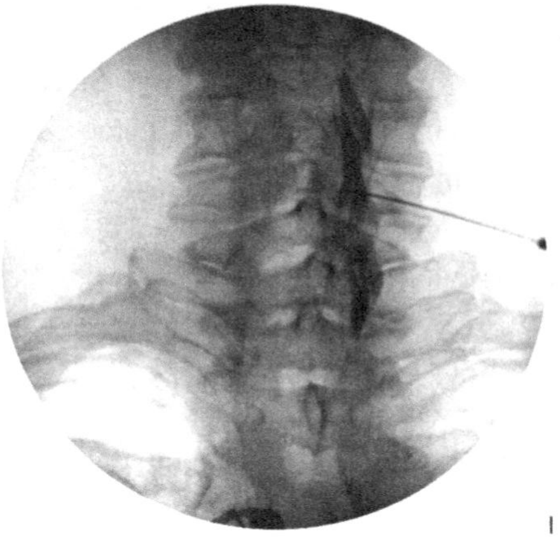

Sample Procedure Note

PREOPERATIVE DIAGNOSIS:	Complex regional pain syndrome (CRPS) upper extremity Limb pain
POSTOPERATIVE DIAGNOSIS:	Same
SURGEON:	_____
ASSISTANT:	_____
TITLE OF PROCEDURE:	Diagnostic _____ stellate ganglion nerve block under fluoroscopic guidance (**Video 7.1**)

https://bcove.video/2rHuBXK

ANESTHESIA:	Monitored anesthesia care
ESTIMATED BLOOD LOSS:	None
COMPLICATIONS:	None
DRAINS:	None
IV FLUID:	200 mL lactated ringer

(continued)

(continued)

Indications: _____-year-old _____ (male/female) complaining of pain in the upper extremity consistent with CRPS. Our plan is to perform a diagnostic stellate ganglion nerve block. The risks and benefits of _____ stellate ganglion nerve block were discussed in detail. The patient understands and accepts that the risks include, but are not limited to, increase in pain, nerve injury, infection, pneumothorax, bleeding, hematoma, paralysis, stroke, and death. Alternatives to nerve blocks, or noninterventional therapy, were discussed and informed consent obtained.

DESCRIPTION OF PROCEDURE
Intravenous access was established. The patient was escorted to the fluoroscopy suite and placed in the supine position. Noninvasive monitoring was applied. Universal Site and Side Protocol was followed and documented. Safe Injection and Infection Control Practices as recommended by the Center for Disease Control, including the use of a face mask, were strictly followed. The neck area is widely prepped using isopropyl alcohol per protocol, and sterile drapes applied. Time-out was performed. Landmarks of the sternal notch, sternocleidomastoid muscle, and longus colli muscle were identified. Using a 25-gauge needle, a skin wheal was raised with 1% lidocaine. A 22-gauge 3.5-inch curved Quincke spinal needle was advanced under fluoroscopic guidance over the lateral border of the _____ vertebral body on the _____ side. Once the vertebral body was in contact, AP and lateral views of the fluoroscope confirmed adequate needle placement. At this point, 2 mL of Omnipaque-240 contrast was injected under live fluoroscopic guidance through a T-Connector extension tubing outlining positive uptake of the stellate ganglion. After negative aspiration for heme, a total volume of 8 mL of .25% bupivacaine was injected through the needle. Once the procedure was completed, all needles were withdrawn from the patient intact. A bandage was applied to the puncture site. The patient tolerated this sequence well, there were no complications noted. The patient was discharged in hemodynamically and neurologically stable condition, with review of postprocedural instructions. We will follow up with the patient in 2 to 4 weeks.

_____
Attending Physician

CELIAC PLEXUS BLOCK

ANATOMY

- The celiac plexus is also known as the solar plexus. It is the largest plexus of the sympathetic nervous system. It is an organized network of nerves, which is located in the retroperitoneal space of the abdomen behind the stomach and the omental bursa. It is formed by the greater and lesser splanchnic nerves bilaterally, and the fibers from the anterior and posterior vagal trunks. The celiac plexus is located at the level of T12–L1.

INDICATIONS

- Pain arising from intra-abdominal structures (esophagus, pancreas, gallbladder, liver mesentery, omentum, spleen, and kidneys)
- Intra-abdominal malignancy (pancreatic cancer)
- Chronic pancreatitis

CONTRAINDICATIONS

- Bleeding and infection risks
- If source of pain is no longer being transmitted through autonomic nerves
- Presence of an aortic aneurysm

TECHNIQUE

- Patient position: the patient is placed in a prone position
- Recommended needle: 22-gauge 7-inch spinal needle
- Medication: 1% lidocaine with epinephrine for test dose and .5% bupivacaine. Steroids may be added for chronic pancreatitis
- Contrast volume recommended: 5 mL
- C-arm positioning: The C-arm is placed over the thoracolumbar junction and then rotated obliquely 20 to 30 degrees until the tip of the transverse process of the L1 overlies the anterolateral margin of the L1 vertebral body.

- Technique

  1. Clean the skin in sterile fashion.

  2. Anesthetize the subcutaneous tissues over the superior margin of the L1 vertebral body with 1 mL to 2 mL of 1% lidocaine.

  3. Since the aorta lies on the left of midline, a left-sided transaortic single-needle technique if often used for the block.

  4. A 22-gauge 7-inch spinal needle is advanced using a coaxial technique caudally to the margin of the 12th rib and cephalad to the transverse process of the L1 and toward the anterolateral margin of the L1 vertebral body.

  5. Rotate the C-arm into a lateral position.

  6. Advance the needle to lie 2 cm to 3 cm anterior to the anterior margin of the L1 vertebral body.

  7. Connect a 20-mL syringe to the spinal needle, and continuously aspirate while advancing the needle anteriorly to the anterior border of the L1.

  8. If the blood appears in the syringe, the needle has gone through the aorta and should continue to advance through the anterior wall of the aorta until the blood is no longer being aspirated.

  9. In the lateral projection, the final needle endpoint is the anterolateral surface of the aorta, approximately 2 cm anterior the vertebral body of L1.

  10. Injection of approximately 2 mL of contrast with live fluoroscopy should highlight the anterior surface of the aorta. With live fluoroscopy, pulsation of the aorta is frequently seen (Figures 7.3 and 7.4).

  11. Rotate the C-arm for AP position.

  12. Final needle position is confirmed by injecting 2 mL to 3 mL of contrast with live fluoroscopy.

  13. If the contrast spreads bilaterally and past midline over the anterior surface of the aorta, a single-needle technique is recommended and injection of the anesthetic can be performed at this time. If the contrast only spreads on the left side, then the same technique can be performed as described earlier for the right side.

COMPLICATIONS

- Severe hypotension
- Diarrhea
- Bleeding due to aorta or inferior vena cava injury by the needle (retroperitoneal hemorrhage)
- Intravascular injection (should be prevented by using contrast to assess needle positioning)
- Upper abdominal organ puncture with abscess or cyst formation
- Paraplegia from injecting into the vessels (artery of Adamkiewicz) that supply the spinal cord (should be prevented by using contrast to assess needle positioning)
- Sexual dysfunction if the injectate spreads to the sympathetic chain bilaterally
- Pneumothorax
- Lumbar nerve root irritation if the injectate spreads toward the lumbar plexus

EXAMPLES

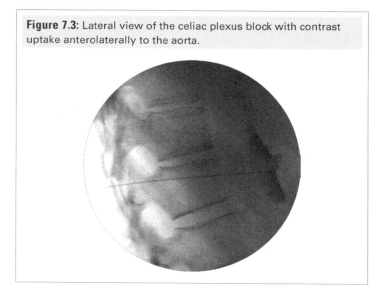

Figure 7.3: Lateral view of the celiac plexus block with contrast uptake anterolaterally to the aorta.

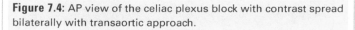

Figure 7.4: AP view of the celiac plexus block with contrast spread bilaterally with transaortic approach.

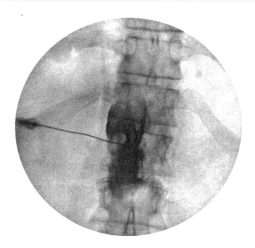

Sample Procedure Note

PREOPERATIVE DIAGNOSIS:	Pancreatic cancer Abdominal pain
POSTOPERATIVE DIAGNOSIS:	Same
SURGEON:	_____
ASSISTANT:	_____
TITLE OF PROCEDURE:	Diagnostic _____ T12/L1 celiac plexus block under fluoroscopic guidance (Video 7.2)

https://bcove.video/2rGugEU

ANESTHESIA:	Monitored anesthesia care
ESTIMATED BLOOD LOSS:	None
COMPLICATIONS:	None
DRAINS:	None
IV FLUID:	200 mL lactated ringer

Indications: _____-year-old _____ (male/female) complaining of pain in the abdomen that is consistent with the innervation

(*continued*)

(continued)

of the celiac plexus. Our plan is to perform a diagnostic T12/L1
celiac plexus block under fluoroscopic guidance today. The
risks and benefits of a celiac plexus block were discussed in
detail. The patient understands and accepts that the risks
include, but are not limited to, increase in pain, nerve injury,
infection, bleeding, hematoma, paralysis, spinal headache, stroke,
pneumothorax, discitis, and death. Alternatives to nerve blocks, or
noninterventional therapy were discussed, and informed consent
obtained.

DESCRIPTION OF PROCEDURE
Intravenous access was established. The patient was escorted
to the fluoroscopy suite and placed in the prone position.
Noninvasive monitoring was applied. Universal Site and Side
Protocol was followed and documented. Safe Injection and
Infection Control Practices as recommended by the Center for
Disease Control, including the use of a face mask, were strictly
followed. The lumbar area is widely prepped using isopropyl
alcohol per protocol, and sterile drapes applied. Time-out was
performed. Using fluoroscopic guidance, the lumbar vertebral
bodies were identified. Using a 25-gauge needle, a skin wheal
was raised with 1% lidocaine. The fluoroscope was obliqued
30 degrees to the _____ with a cephalocaudal tilt to align the
vertebral endplates and outline the landmark of the Scotty
dog. A 22-gauge 7-inch curved Quincke spinal needle was
placed at the junction where the transverse process meets the
vertebral body at the T12/L1 on the _____ vertebral body. The
needle was independently carried down to the anterolateral
portion of the vertebral body under fluoroscopic guidance.
Once the anterolateral portion of vertebral body was in contact,
continuous aspiration was used to identify the aorta. Once
aortic blood was aspirated, the needle was advanced until blood
was no longer aspirated from the needle. At this point, AP
and lateral projections of the fluoroscope confirmed adequate
needle placement. At this time, 2 mL of Omnipaque-240
contrast was injected under live fluoroscopic guidance through
a T-Connector extension tubing outlining a positive neurogram
of the celiac plexus. There was no evidence of intrathecal or

(continued)

(*continued*)

intravascular spread. After negative aspiration for heme and cerebrospinal fluid (CSF), 20 mL of .25% preservative-free bupivacaine was injected without complication. Once the procedure was completed, all needles were withdrawn from the patient intact. A bandage was applied to the puncture site. The patient tolerated this procedure well, there were no complications noted. The patient was discharged home in hemodynamically and neurologically stable condition, with review of post procedural instructions.

_____

Attending Physician

LUMBAR SYMPATHETIC BLOCK

ANATOMY

- The preganglionic nerve fibers of the sympathetic nervous system are located in the intermediolateral cell column from T11 to L2. These preganglionic fibers then exit along with a nerve root and synapse with the postganglionic sympathetic fibers.

INDICATIONS

- CRPS Type I and II of lower extremities
- Peripheral vascular disease
- Raynaud's phenomenon
- Trench foot
- Postsurgical leg pain
- Neuropathic pain of lower extremities
- Postherpetic neuralgia of lower extremities
- Phantom limb pain
- Hyperhidrosis

CONTRAINDICATIONS

- Bleeding and infection risks
- Patient refusal

TECHNIQUE

- Patient position: prone with a pillow under the lower abdomen to reduce the lumbar lordosis on the C-arm table
- C-arm position: center the C-arm over the mid-lumbar region and then ipsilaterally oblique 25 to 30 degrees until the tip of the transverse process of L3 overlies the anterolateral margin of L3 vertebral body.
- Recommended needle: 22-gauge 5- to 7-inch spinal needle
- Medication: 15 mL to 20 mL of .25% bupivacaine
- Contrast volume recommended
- Technique:
  1. Clean the skin in sterile fashion.
  2. Anesthetize the skin and subcutaneous tissues over the anterolateral surface of the L3 vertebral body with 2 mL to 3 mL of 1% lidocaine.
  3. Advance the spinal needle using a coaxial technique toward the anterolateral surface of the L3 vertebral body with utilization of intermittent fluoroscopy.
  4. The needle tip should be kept by the lateral margin of the vertebral body until the needle contacts bone.
  5. The needle is then walked off the bone laterally.
  6. Rotate the C-arm laterally.
  7. Advance the needle until the needle tip is over the anterior one third of the vertebral body.
  8. Inject 1 mL to 2 mL of contrast to confirm depth (Figures 7.5 and 7.6).
  9. Rotate the C-arm in AP position.
  10. Verify the needle tip is medial to the lateral margin of the vertebral body.
  11. After negative aspiration for heme or CSF, injection of the local anesthesia (15 mL–20 mL of .25% bupivacaine) may be performed in increments of 5 mL and intermittent negative aspirations.
  12. Monitor the changes of skin temperature to assess for successful blockade.

COMPLICATIONS

- Orthostatic hypotension
- Damage to ilioinguinal or genitofemoral nerve
- Hematuria due to kidney trauma
- Spinal nerve, epidural, or intrathecal injection

EXAMPLES

Figure 7.5: Lateral radiograph indicating the endpoint slightly anterolateral to the L3 vertebral body.

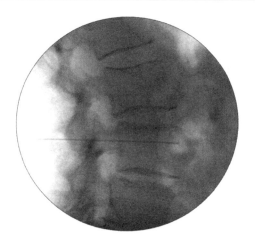

Figure 7.6: AP radiograph with contrast uptake of the lumbar sympathetic plexus.

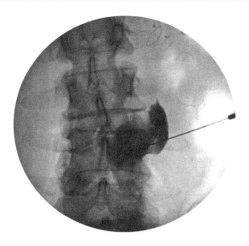

Sample Procedure Note

PREOPERATIVE DIAGNOSIS:	CRPS type _____ lower extremity Limb pain
POSTOPERATIVE DIAGNOSIS:	Same
SURGEON:	_____
ASSISTANT:	_____
TITLE OF PROCEDURE:	Diagnostic _____ lumbar Sympathetic block under fluoroscopic guidance (Video 7.3)

https://bcove.video/2wAloFA

ANESTHESIA:	Monitored anesthesia care
ESTIMATED BLOOD LOSS:	None
COMPLICATIONS:	None
DRAINS:	None
IV FLUID:	200 mL lactated ringer

Indications: _____-year-old _____ (male/female) complaining of pain in the lower extremity that is consistent with CRPS. Our plan is to perform a diagnostic lumbar sympathetic block under fluoroscopic guidance today. The risks and benefits of _____ a lumbar sympathetic block were discussed in detail. The patient understands and accepts that the risks include, but are not limited to, increase in pain, nerve injury, infection, bleeding, hematoma, paralysis, spinal headache, stroke, discitis, and death. Alternatives to nerve blocks, or noninterventional therapy, were discussed and informed consent obtained.

DESCRIPTION OF PROCEDURE
Intravenous access was established. The patient was escorted to the fluoroscopy suite and placed in the prone position. Noninvasive monitoring was applied. Universal Site and Side Protocol was followed and documented. Safe Injection and Infection Control Practices as recommended by the Center for Disease Control, including the use of a face mask, were

(continued)

(continued)

strictly followed. The lumbar area is widely prepped using isopropyl alcohol per protocol, and sterile drapes applied. Time-out was performed. Using fluoroscopic guidance, the lumbar vertebral bodies were identified. Using a 25-gauge needle, a skin wheal was raised with 1% lidocaine. The fluoroscope was obliqued 30 degrees to the _____ with a cephalocaudal tilt to align the vertebral endplates and outline the landmark of the Scotty dog. A 22-gauge 5-inch curved Quincke spinal needle was placed at the junction where the transverse process meets the vertebral body at the _____ vertebral body. The needle was independently carried down to the anterolateral portion of the vertebral body under fluoroscopic guidance. AP and lateral projections of the fluoroscope confirmed adequate needle placement. At this time, 2 mL of Omnipaque-240 contrast was injected under live fluoroscopic guidance through a T-Connector extension tubing outlining a positive neurogram of the lumbar sympathetic ganglion. There was no evidence of intrathecal or intravascular spread. After negative aspiration for heme and CSF, 20 mL of .25% preservative-free bupivacaine was injected without complication. Once the procedure was completed, all needles were withdrawn from the patient intact. A bandage was applied to the puncture site. The patient tolerated this procedure well, there were no complications noted. The patient was discharged in hemodynamically and neurologically stable condition, with review of postprocedural instructions.

Plan: If the patient received 50% or greater improvement of their pain, we will repeat the procedure in 2 to 4 weeks' time. If today's injection does not alleviate the patient's pain by 50%, we will perform a diagnostic lumbar sympathetic block at a different level of the lumbar sympathetic chain under fluoroscopic guidance in 2 to 3 weeks.

_____

Attending Physician

SUPERIOR HYPOGASTRIC BLOCK

ANATOMY

- The superior hypogastric plexus is formed from the two lower lumbar splanchnic nerves (L3–L4), which are branches of the chain ganglia. The plexus also contains parasympathetic fibers formed from the pelvic splanchnic nerve (S2–S4) and ascend from the inferior hypogastric plexus. The plexus is located retroperitoneally and lies anteriorly to the fourth and fifth lumbar and sacral vertebrae. Sympathetic nerves which pass through the plexus nerve innervate the pelvic organs, including bladder, uterus, vagina, rectum, and prostate.

INDICATIONS

- Pelvic visceral pain or pelvic cancer
- Malignant or nonmalignant origin pain in the proximal vagina, ovaries, uterus, prostate, and rectum
- Sympathetically mediated pain of the hypogastric region (CRPS)
- Pelvic fibrosis
- Pelvis neurodystonica
- Pelvic inflammatory disease
- Endometriosis
- Interstitial cystitis
- Prostatitis
- Refractory penile pain
- Dysmenorrhea and dyspareunia
- Vulvitis
- Cystitis
- Pelvic radiation-induced neuropathy
- Irritable bowel syndrome
- Painful pelvic adhesions resulting from abdominal or gynecological surgeries

CONTRAINDICATIONS

- Systemic or local infection in the area of the injection
- Coagulopathy
- Patient refusal

TECHNIQUE

- Patient position: Patient lies prone with a pillow under the lower abdomen to reduce the lumbar lordosis
- C-arm position: Oblique approximately 25 to 35 degrees with a 20 to 25 degree cephalad tilt to allow L5/S1 disc visualization
- Recommended needle: 22-gauge 5- to 7-inch needle
- Medication: 8 mL to 10 mL of local anesthetic (e.g., .25% bupivacaine)
- Contrast volume recommended: 2 mL to 3 mL
- Technique:
  1. Prep the skin in sterile fashion.
  2. Oblique the C-arm 25 to 35 degrees ipsilaterally with 25 to 35 degrees of cephalad tilt.
  3. Identify a small triangular window bounded superiorly by the L5 transverse process, laterally by the iliac crest, and medially the L5/S1 facet joint and superior articular process of S1.
  4. Anesthetize the skin over this small triangular window with 1% lidocaine.
  5. Advance the 22-gauge spinal needle through the small triangular window with intermittent fluoroscopy. The trajectory of the needle advancement involves transdiscal approach through the L5/S1 disc to approach the anterolateral surface of the vertebral column at L5/S1 level.
  6. Tilt the C-arm laterally and advance the needle to position over the anterolateral surface of the lumbosacral junction. The endpoint is when the needles are aligned with the anterior vertebral margin in the lateral position.
  7. Place the C-arm in the AP position.
  8. Inject a small amount of contrast (2 mL–3 mL) and confirm spread along the anterior aspect of the lumbosacral junction (Figures 7.7, 7.8, and 7.9).
  9. A contralateral procedure may be performed.
  10. Inject 8 mL to 10 mL of .25% bupivacaine.

COMPLICATIONS

- Intravascular injection of neurolytic solution
- In bilateral, male sexual dysfunction may occur

EXAMPLES

Figure 7.7: Lateral radiograph outlining contrast uptake of the superior hypogastric plexus.

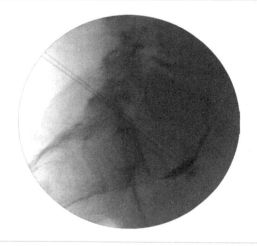

Figure 7.8: AP view of the right side contrast uptake of the superior hypogastric plexus.

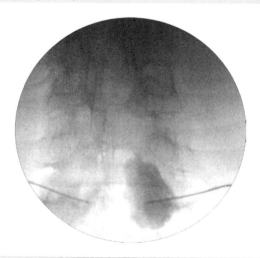

Figure 7.9: AP view of the left side contrast uptake of the superior hypogastric plexus.

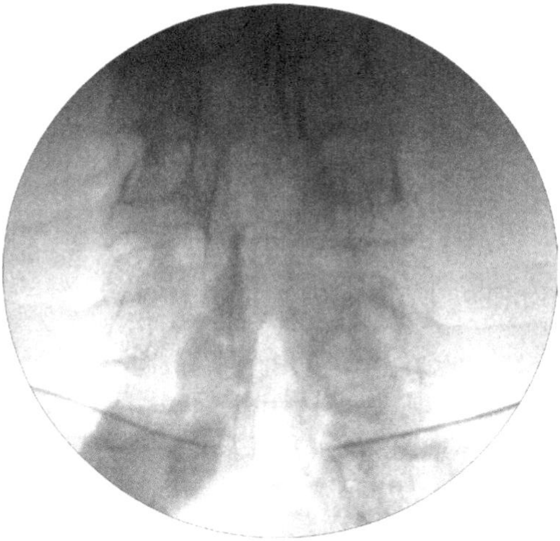

Sample Procedure Note

PREOPERATIVE DIAGNOSIS:	Pelvic pain Abdominal pain
POSTOPERATIVE DIAGNOSIS:	Same
SURGEON:	_____
ASSISTANT:	_____
TITLE OF PROCEDURE:	Diagnostic _____ L5/S1 hypogastric plexus block under fluoroscopic guidance
ANESTHESIA:	Monitored anesthesia care
ESTIMATED BLOOD LOSS:	None
COMPLICATIONS:	None
DRAINS:	None
IV FLUID:	200 mL lactated ringer

(*continued*)

(*continued*)

Indications: _____-year-old _____ (male/female) complaining
of pain in the pelvis and lower abdomen that is consistent with
the innervation of the hypogastric plexus. Our plan is to perform
a diagnostic L5/S1 hypogastric plexus block under fluoroscopic
guidance today. The risks and benefits of a hypogastric plexus
block were discussed in detail. The patient understands and
accepts that the risks include, but are not limited to, increase in
pain, nerve injury, infection, bleeding, hematoma, paralysis, spinal
headache, stroke, discitis, and death. Alternatives to nerve blocks,
or noninterventional therapy, were discussed and informed
consent obtained.

DESCRIPTION OF PROCEDURE
Intravenous access was established. The patient was escorted
to the fluoroscopy suite and placed in the prone position.
Noninvasive monitoring was applied. Universal Site and Side
Protocol was followed and documented. Safe Injection and
Infection Control Practices as recommended by the Center
for Disease Control, including the use of a face mask, were
strictly followed. The lumbar area is widely prepped using
isopropyl alcohol per protocol, and sterile drapes applied.
Time-out was performed. Using fluoroscopic guidance the
lumbar vertebral bodies were identified. Using a 25-gauge needle,
a skin wheal was raised with 1% lidocaine. The fluoroscope was
obliqued 30 degrees to the _____ with a cephalocaudal tilt to
align the vertebral endplates and outline the landmark of the
Scotty dog. A 22-gauge 7-inch curved Quincke spinal needle
was placed just lateral to the midpoint of the superior articular
process of the L5/S1 level on the _____ . The needle was guided
transdiscal under fluoroscopic guidance. At this point, the needle
was independently carried down to the anterolateral portion
of the vertebral body under fluoroscopic guidance. Once the
anterolateral portion of vertebral body was in contact, 2 mL of
Omnipaque-240 contrast was injected under live fluoroscopic
guidance through a T-Connector extension tubing outlining
a positive neurogram of the hypogastric plexus. There was no
evidence of intrathecal or intravascular spread. After negative

(*continued*)

(*continued*)

> aspiration for heme and CSF, 20 mL of .25% preservative-free bupivacaine was injected without complication. Once the procedure was completed, all needles were withdrawn from the patient intact. A bandage was applied to the puncture site. The patient tolerated this procedure well, there were no complications noted. The patient was discharged in hemodynamically and neurologically stable condition, with review of postprocedural instructions.
>
> _____
> **Attending Physician**

GANGLION IMPAR BLOCK

ANATOMY

- The ganglion impar (also known as the ganglion of Walther) is located at the end of the sympathetic chain in the pelvis. It is situated anteriorly to the sacrococcygeal junction. It provides visceral afferents from the perineum, anus, rectum, distal urethra, and distal ⅓ of the vagina.

INDICATIONS

- Sympathetically mediated pain in the pelvic region
- Perineal pain
- Intrapelvic pathology
- Postsurgical pelvic pain
- Postradiation pelvic pain
- Chronic prostatitis
- Proctalgia fugax
- Coccydynia
- Endometriosis
- Scrotal pain
- Vaginal protrusion
- Distal urethral pain

CONTRAINDICATIONS

- Systemic or local infection in the area of the injection
- Coagulopathy
- Patient refusal

TECHNIQUE

- Patient position: Patient lies prone
- C-arm position: Lateral and AP views
- Recommended needle: 22-gauge short-beveled 3-inch needle or 5-inch spinal needle
- Medication: 8 mL to 10 mL of .25% bupivacaine
- Contrast volume recommended: 3 mL to 4 mL
- Technique:
  1. Prep the skin in sterile fashion
  2. Place the C-arm in the lateral position
  3. Identify the sacral spinous process, the sacrum, the ischial spine, and the sacrococcygeal joint
  4. Anesthetize the skin over the sacrococcygeal joint with 1% lidocaine
  5. Advance the needle with intermittent fluoroscopy through the sacrococcygeal joint until a subtle loss of resistance is felt when the needle tip passes through the anterior sacrococcygeal ligament
  6. Confirm the needle tip is anterior to the anterior coccygeal line
  7. Inject 1 mL to 2 mL of contrast is dorsal to the rectal gas and anterior to the coccyx
  8. Rotate the C-arm into the AP position
  9. With live fluoroscopy, inject 1 mL to 2 mL of contrast to confirm contrast flow to be midline (Figures 7.10 and 7.11)
  10. Inject 8 mL to 10 mL of .25% bupivacaine

COMPLICATIONS

- Perforation of the rectum
- Infection
- Intravascular injection
- Internal bleeding

EXAMPLES

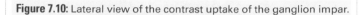

Figure 7.10: Lateral view of the contrast uptake of the ganglion impar.

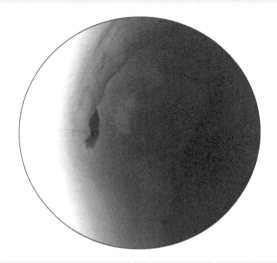

Figure 7.11: AP view of the contrast uptake of the ganglion impar.

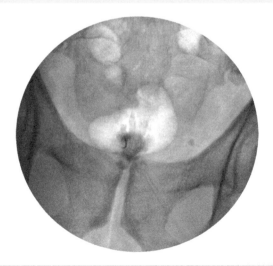

Sample Procedure Note

PREOPERATIVE DIAGNOSIS: Rectal pain
                               Low back pain
POSTOPERATIVE DIAGNOSIS: Same
SURGEON: _____
ASSISTANT: _____
TITLE OF PROCEDURE: Ganglion impar block
                               under fluoroscopic
                               guidance (**Video 7.4**)

https://bcove.video/2rGuXy5

ANESTHESIA: Monitored anesthesia care
ESTIMATED BLOOD LOSS: None
COMPLICATIONS: None
DRAINS: None
IV FLUID: 200 mL lactated ringer

Indications: _____-year-old _____ (male/female) complaining of
low back pain and pain over the rectum and tailbone. Our plan is to
perform a ganglion impar block under fluoroscopic guidance today.
The risks and benefits of a ganglion impar block were discussed in
detail. The patient understands and accepts that the risks include,
but are not limited to, increase in pain, nerve injury, infection,
bleeding, hematoma, paralysis, spinal headache, stroke, discitis, and
death. Alternatives to nerve blocks, or noninterventional therapy,
were discussed and informed consent obtained.

DESCRIPTION OF PROCEDURE
Intravenous access was established. The patient was escorted
to the fluoroscopy suite and placed in the prone position.
Noninvasive monitoring was applied. Universal Site and Side
Protocol was followed and documented. Safe Injection and
Infection Control Practices as recommended by the Center
for Disease Control, including the use of a face mask, were
strictly followed. The lumbosacral, buttock, and tailbone
area is widely prepped using isopropyl alcohol per protocol,
and sterile drapes applied. Time-out was performed. Using
fluoroscopic guidance the sacrum, coccyx, and caudal canal
was easily identified. Using a 25-gauge needle, a skin wheal
was raised with 1% lidocaine. Under fluoroscopic guidance
in the AP and lateral views, a 22-gauge Quincke needle was

(continued)

(continued)

placed through the sacrococcygeal ligament anterior to the coccyx where the ganglion impar resides without difficulty. AP and lateral projections of the fluoroscope confirmed adequate needle placement. At this point, 2 mL of Omnipaque-240 contrast was injected under live fluoroscopic guidance outlining a positive neurogram. There was no evidence of intrathecal or intravascular spread. After negative aspiration for heme, CSF, and stool 40 mg of Kenalog with _____mL of .25% preservative-free bupivacaine was injected without complication. Once the procedure was completed all needles were withdrawn from the patient intact. A bandage was applied to the puncture site. The patient tolerated this procedure well, there were no complications noted. The patient was discharged in hemodynamically and neurologically stable condition, with review of postprocedural instructions.

Plan: If the patient received 50% or greater improvement of their pain, we will repeat the procedure in 2 to 4 weeks' time. If today's injection does not alleviate the patient's pain by 50%, we will perform and caudal epidural steroid injection under fluoroscopic guidance.

_____
Attending Physician

COMPLEX REGIONAL PAIN SYNDROME

DEFINITION

- CRPS is defined by the International Association for the Study of Pain as "a variety of painful conditions following injury which appears regionally having a distal predominance of abnormal findings, exceeding in both magnitude and duration of the expected clinical course of the inciting event often resulting in significant impairment of motor function and showing variable progression over time." It was previously referred to as reflex sympathetic dystrophy (RSD) or causalgia and described as a neuropathic pain state with symptoms out of proportion to the initial trauma. It is commonly associated with autonomic dys-regulation, swelling, motor dysfunction, and trophic changes.

ETIOLOGY

- Typically develops after an acute trauma (fractures, sprains, surgeries, crush injury) or after physical stress (stroke, infection, burns, etc.).
- Currently, there is no evidence that any particular or specific injury that occurs regularly manifests as CRPS or that the severity of the injury is related to the development of CRPS.

HISTORY

- Most common complains in CRPS patients include hyperesthesia and/or allodynia.
- Patients with CRPS often describe pain as burning, hot, and achy which may or may not follow a dermatomal distribution.
- Stressors, limb movement, or physical activity can often make the pain worse.
- CRPS is a clinical diagnosis, and the Budapest criteria are frequently used to diagnose CRPS. The patient must report at least one symptom in three of the four following categories:

THE IASP-PROPOSED REVISED CRPS CLINICAL DIAGNOSTIC BUDAPEST CRITERIA:	
Sensory	Hyperesthesia and/or allodynia
Vasomotor	Temperature asymmetry and/or skin color changes and/or skin color asymmetry
Sudomotor/edema	Edema and/or sweating changes and/or sweating asymmetry
Motor/trophic	Decreased range of motion and/or motor dysfunction (weakness, tremor, dystonia) and/or trophic changes
MUST DISPLAY AT LEAST ONE SIGN OR SYMPTOM AT THE TIME OF EVALUATION IN TWO OR MORE OF THE FOLLOWING CATEGORIES:	
Sensory	Evidence of hyperalgesia and/or allodynia (to light touch or deep somatic pressure and/or joint movement)

Vasomotor	Evidence of temperature asymmetry and/or skin color changes and/or asymmetry
Sudomotor/edema	Evidence of decreased range of motion and/or motor dysfunction (weakness, tremor, dystonia) and/or trophic changes (hair, nail, and skin)

PHYSICAL EXAMINATION

- Examination includes objective findings in two out of four of the previous categories. Examination tools include temperature measurement and sensory signs through light touch and pinprick.
- Light touch should be performed with a soft brush or cotton tip. Motor changes may be observed with reduced range of motion and/or tremors.
- Trophic changes may be evident with loss of hair and nail changes.
- Vasomotor signs may be evident by assessing skin color and measuring skin temperature between affected and contralateral unaffected area.
- Severity can be indicated by loss of range of motion, presence of adhesive capsulitis, and muscle atrophy.

DIAGNOSTIC STUDIES

- X-rays may reveal periarticular patchy osteopenia or osteoporosis of the affected area but have low sensitivity. It may also reveal subperiosteal bone resorption.
- MRI may be performed to evaluate for an injury, may reveal soft-tissue edema and enhancement, and skin thickening. It may also reveal patchy subcortical bone marrow edema.
- Triple phase bone scans may reveal increased uptake in all three phases. Increased juxta-articular activity may be seen around all joints of the affected region.

TREATMENT

- Physical therapy (PT) and occupational therapy (OT) objectives include improve range of motion, desensitization therapy, minimal swelling, prevent contracture formation, decrease muscle guarding, and improve function.

- Other nonintervention and nonpharmacological treatments include mirror box therapy, transcutaneous electrical nerve stimulation (TENS) unit, and cognitive behavioral therapy.
- Pharmacological treatment include:
  1. Gabapentin, lyrica, topiramate to help with the neuropathic pain component.
  2. Bisphosphonates help reduce osteoclastic activity and modify inflammatory cytokines.
  3. Calcitonin helps increase intracellular calcium within the dorsal horn.
  4. Ketamine infusion helps by working blocking N-methyl-D-aspartate (NMDA) receptor and thus reducing central sensitization.
- Interventional treatments:
  1. Sympathetic blocks can be used for both diagnostic and therapeutic purposes depending on the location of CRPS.
  2. Radiofrequency sympathectomy may be performed if the diagnostic sympathetic blocks provide short-term relief.
  3. Spinal cord stimulation by stimulating the dorsal column may help modulate the neuropathic pain.

List of Videos

 Video 7.1 Stellate Ganglion Block

https://bcove.video/2rHuBXK

Video 7.2 Transaortic Celiac Plexus Block

https://bcove.video/2rGugEU

 Video 7.3 Lumbar Sympathetic Block

https://bcove.video/2wAloFA

Video 7.4 Ganglion Impar Block

https://bcove.video/2rGuXy5

Spinal Cord Stimulation

Spinal cord stimulators are a type of spinal neuromodulation analgesic system, which is an option for chronic pain that can arise after nerve or nervous system injury. Spinal cord stimulation is a minimally invasive and reversible treatment option that is typically percutaneously or surgically implantation of electrodes into the epidural space after an appropriately conducted temporary screening trial with an external pulse generator to assess the therapeutic efficacy and adverse effects.

MECHANISM OF ACTION

Initially, the spinal cord stimulation was thought to provide analgesia through the gate control theory in the dorsal horn of the spinal cord. The substantia gelatinosa in the dorsal horn is the gate system where pain is modulated. The small painful A-delta and C fibers and large (A-beta) nerve fibers synapse at the gate. The large fiber activation then inhibited the painful small fibers and thus, closing the gate and providing pain relief. Newer theories indicate that spinal cord stimulation provides relief of neuropathic pain in part by the wide dynamic range neuron suppression in the dorsal horn.

Pain relief from the spinal cord stimulation may take days to weeks after stimulation has been turned on indicating a central mechanism of analgesia.

INDICATIONS

Typically, spinal cord stimulation is considered for patients with chronic pain who have failed conservative approaches. Some common indications for spinal cord stimulation include the following:

1. Failed back surgery syndrome: Involves placement of electrodes into the epidural space adjacent to the spinal area, which is thought to be the source of the pain. An electric current is then applied to achieve neuromodulatory effects.
2. Refractory radiculitis in the upper or lower extremity
3. Complex regional pain syndrome: Spinal cord stimulation may be helpful if conventional therapies treatment options fail.
4. HIV polyneuropathy, painful diabetic neuropathy refractory to conventional treatment options
5. Pain from epidural fibrosis
6. Pain from arachnoiditis
7. In Europe, intractable angina and peripheral vascular disease are common indications for spinal cord stimulation.

SCREENING

PSYCHOLOGICAL SCREENING: Performed prior to spinal cord stimulator trial and may be required by insurance companies for approval. High levels of depression, anxiety, coping, and somatization and hypochondriasis are associated with worse outcomes after spinal cord stimulation. Treatment of any psychological condition may be warranted prior to proceeding with spinal cord stimulation.

IMAGING STUDIES: Spine imaging studies should be reviewed to assess technical difficulty.

PACEMAKERS: In patients with cardiac pacemaker and internal defibrillators, spinal cord stimulator compatibility should be established prior to the stimulator trial. Newer pacemakers have minimal interaction if strict bipolar right ventricular sensing is used. Patients with defibrillators require closer observation to ensure stimulation does not result in defibrillator discharges. A cardiology consultation should take place as a part of preprocedure evaluation.

DURATION OF PAIN: Spinal cord stimulation is more likely to be effective if placed less than 2 to 3 years from the onset of pain and less effective if delay is greater than 6 to 7 years from the onset of pain.

EQUIPMENT

IMPLANTABLE PULSE GENERATORS: Deliver electrical stimulation that can be modified by altering the pulse width, frequency, and amplitude which allows pain suppression.

1. Frequency: Standard spinal cord stimulation delivers stimulation at relatively low frequency (around 50 Hz). Newer high-frequency (HF-10) generators use a biphasic stimulator wave with pulse width of approximately 30 seconds at the rate of 10,000 Hz. These high-frequency stimulators do not cause paresthesias. The new high-frequency stimulator leads are typically placed based on the location of the pain, usually with one lead tip at the top of T8 and the other on the top of T9 to capture low back pain and leg pain. Generally, patient feedback is not required for high-frequency stimulator placement during trial and implantation.

2. Burst stimulation is a new form of spinal cord stimulation that consists of five high-frequency burst spikes at a rate of 40 Hz with a pulse width of 1 microsecond. Burst stimulation is not likely to cause paresthesias and may provide better reduction to neuropathic pain when compared to standard tonic stimulation.

LEADS

1. Surgical paddle leads are flat-shaped leads which have two to five columns of electrodes. The paddle leads provide unidirectional stimulation toward the spinal cord, and allows for a deeper penetration of the electrical stimulus. However, they are bulkier and should be avoided in areas of spinal stenosis.

2. Percutaneous cylindrical leads can be placed through a 14-gauge epidural needle, and transmit current circumferentially. If necessary, these are easily removed. The most common complication is lead migration that may occur during early postprocedure.

3. Percutaneous paddle leads: New entry system that allows insertion of multiple leads percutaneously, including an S-series paddle lead, at the level of L1 or below.

PROGRAMMERS

1. Usually, the patient is provided a handheld programmer with settings determined by stimulation which provides the best relief of the patient's pain. The patient typically can chose between these programmed settings.

PROCEDURE PLANNING

Both the trial and implantation are performed with fluoroscopy and are typically outpatient procedures. Both procedures require strict sterile techniques, with full skin preparation and draping, and preprocedure administration of antibiotics.

The level for lead position depends on the location of the pain. The usual levels for lead position for pain are the following:

LEAD PLACEMENT LEVELS	INDICATIONS
C2, C3	Occipital neuralgia, cervical postlaminectomy syndrome, axial neck pain
C4	Shoulder joint pain
C5, C6	Upper extremity: arm and hand pain, peripheral neuropathy involving upper extremities
C7	Hands, complex regional pain syndrome I/II
T2, T3	Angina
T4, T5	Postmastectomy pain syndrome, postthoracotomy pain syndrome, postherpetic neuralgia
T6, T7	Chronic intractable abdominal pain, chronic pancreatitis

(continued)

(*continued*)

T8, T9	Low back pain, lumbar postlaminectomy syndrome, axial low back pain
T10, T11	Lumbar radiculopathy, restless leg syndrome
T12	Hip pain, groin pain
S2	Urogenital pain, rectum, inguinal neuralgia, posthernia repair pain
S3	Vulvodynia, endometriosis

TRIAL DURATION: Average trial duration lasts from 4 to 10 days. The trial duration may need to be adjusted based on patient profile, such as patients who are on anticoagulation or antiplatelet medication for other comorbidities.

The trial is considered successful and implantation is recommended when the trial results in more than 50% pain reduction with improved functionality.

TRIAL TECHNIQUE

a. Patient positioning: Patient is placed in a prone position with lumbar support to reduce the lumbar lordosis.

b. The area is prepped and draped in sterile fashion.

c. The skin is localized with 1% lidocaine with epinephrine.

d. A 14-gauge needle is then introduced percutaneously at the medial border of the pedicle at one to two vertebral bodies below the desired entry site in an acute angle to allow for a gradual entry into the epidural space using a paramedian walk-off approach that will ensure appropriate epidural entry.

e. Advance the needle with intermittent fluoroscopy in the anteroposterior (AP) view with the needle at a 30-degree or more shallow angle.

f. The epidural access is achieved by utilizing the "loss of resistance" technique with air or saline described in Chapters 4–6.

g. A lateral fluoroscopic image is then obtained to visualize the depth of the epidural space.

h. Once a reliable dorsal epidural space entry is achieved, the lead is introduced and advanced with intermittent fluoroscopy (Figures 8.1 and 8.4).

i. Once the lead(s) is in position, stimulation testing is performed (if required) (Figures 8.2 and 8.3).

j. Once the testing is complete, the stylets are removed and the leads are secured (suture, adhesive bandage, or via the supplied anchors) with frequent fluoroscopic confirmation that the leads have not migrated.

k. When in the recovery room, the external remote is connected and the patient is instructed to continue his or her daily activities.

COMPLICATIONS

a. Lead migration

b. Lead fracture

c. Seroma formation

d. Infection

e. Dural puncture/postdural puncture headache

f. Epidural hematoma (emergency)

g. Spinal cord trauma

h. Nerve Injury

CURRENT COMPANIES OFFERING SPINAL CORD STIMULATION

a. Medtronic

b. St. Jude Medical

c. Boston Scientific

d. Nevro

e. Nuvectra

f. Stimwave

EXAMPLES

Figure 8.1: Lateral view of the cervical spinal cord stimulator trial.

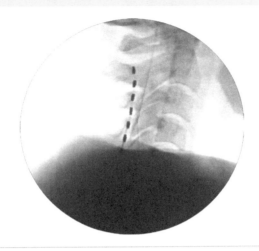

Figure 8.2: AP view of the of the cervical spinal cord stimulator trial.

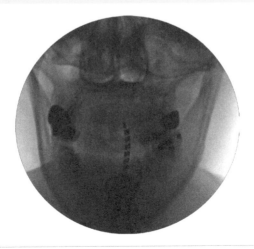

Figure 8.3: AP view of the of the lumbar spinal cord stimulator trial.

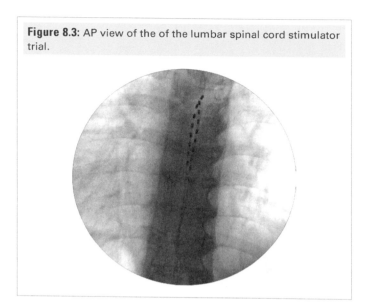

Figure 8.4: Lateral view of the lumbar spinal cord stimulator trial.

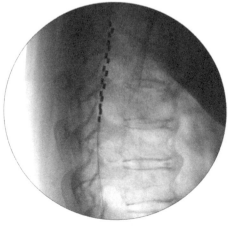

Sample Procedure Note

PREOPERATIVE DIAGNOSIS:	Lumbar radiculitis Lumbar disc displacement Low back pain
POSTOPERATIVE DIAGNOSIS:	Same
SURGEON:	_____
ASSISTANT:	_____
TITLE OF PROCEDURE:	Percutaneous spinal cord stimulator trial, _____ Octrode electrode placement in the epidural space in the _____ region under fluoroscopic guidance

https://bcove.video/2wKXreG

https://bcove.video/2rFlW8g

Analysis and reprogramming of stimulator (**Videos 8.1 and 8.2**)

ANESTHESIA:	Monitored anesthesia care
PRE-OP ANTIBIOTICS:	_____
ESTIMATED BLOOD LOSS:	None
COMPLICATIONS:	None
DRAINS:	None
IV FLUID	500 mL lactated ringer
PREOPERATIVE ANTIBIOTIC	_____

IV, intravenous.

Indications: _____-year-old _____ (male/female) complaining of _____ pain that radiates to the _____. The patient has tried conservative treatment and management including, but not limited to, interventional injections, physical therapy, rest, ice, heat, and oral medication management with minimal improvement of the pain. Our plan is to perform a spinal cord stimulator trial under fluoroscopic guidance today. The risks and benefits of _____ spinal cord stimulator trial were discussed in detail. The patient understands and accepts that the risks include, but are not limited to, increase in pain, nerve injury, infection, bleeding, hematoma, paralysis, spinal headache, stroke,

(continued)

(continued)

discitis, and death. Alternatives to the spinal cord stimulator, or noninterventional therapy, were discussed and informed consent obtained.

DESCRIPTION OF PROCEDURE
Intravenous access was established. The patient was escorted to the fluoroscopy suite and placed in the prone position. Noninvasive monitoring was applied. Universal Site and Side Protocol was followed and documented. Safe Injection and Infection Control Practices as recommended by the Center for Disease Control, including the use of a face mask, were strictly followed. The lumbar area is widely prepped using chlorhexidine × 3 and isopropyl alcohol × 3 per protocol. A full body thyroid drape was used along with Ioban for sterile properties. A sterile drape/cover was placed over the C-arm. Time-out was performed. The vertebral endplates were aligned. Using fluoroscopic guidance the lumbar vertebral bodies, spinous process, pedicles, and disc spaces were identified. _____ mL of _____ local anesthetic was infiltrated into the skin and deeper tissue using a 25-gauge needle. Under fluoroscopic guidance, a 14-gauge Tuohy needle was placed midway between the spinous process and the pedicle of the _____ vertebral body on the_____ side. Using a 45- to 60-degree angle, each needle was independently carried down to the epidural space at _____ under fluoroscopic guidance. Intermittent loss of resistance technique with saline was used to identify the epidural space. Once the epidural space was identified, AP and lateral projections of the fluoroscope confirmed adequate needle placement. At this time, a 45-cm Octrode lead was threaded through the Tuohy needle in the cephalad direction maintaining midline position and the posterior position of the epidural space. The leads were threaded up the _____ level. There was no cerebrospinal fluid (CSF) or heme at any time. At this point, the patient was awoken from monitored anesthesia care (MAC) and the leads were tested with the company representative. We were able to achieve pain/paresthesia overlap over the dermatomal segments of the patient's pain. At this point, the needles and stylets were removed intact without difficulty. The spinal cord stimulator leads were secured to the skin with 0 silk suture, sterile strips, mastisol, and tegaderm. The patient

(continued)

(continued)

tolerated this procedure well, there were no complications noted. The patient was transported to the postanesthesia care unit (PACU) and was programmed with the representative. Once all programming was complete, the patient was discharged in hemodynamically and neurologically stable condition, with review of postprocedural instructions.

Plan: We will perform a 5-day trial with the spinal cord stimulator. If the patient received 50% or greater improvement of their pain along with improved function of activity of daily living, we will plan on permanent implantation of the spinal cord stimulator system.

_____

Attending Physician

List of Videos

 Video 8.1 Cervical Spinal Cord Stimulator Trial

https://bcove.video/2wKXreG

Video 8.2 Thoracolumbar Spinal Cord Stimulator Trial

https://bcove.video/2rFlW8g

Bonus Videos: Other Commonly Performed Procedures

9

Trigeminal Nerve Block

- Indications: Treatment of trigeminal neuralgia, herpes zoster ophthalmicus, postherpetic neuralgia, facial pain

Sample Procedure Note

PREOPERATIVE DIAGNOSIS: Trigeminal neuralgia
Facial pain

POSTOPERATIVE DIAGNOSIS: Same

SURGEON: _____

ASSISTANT: _____

TITLE OF PROCEDURE: Diagnostic _____ trigeminal nerve block under fluoroscopic guidance (**Video 9.1**)

https://bcove.video/2jTZcwU

ANESTHESIA: Local anesthesia

ESTIMATED BLOOD LOSS: None

COMPLICATIONS: None

Indications: _____ year-old (male/female) complaining of facial pain over the trigeminal nerve distribution. Our plan is to perform a diagnostic trigeminal nerve block under fluoroscopic guidance. The risks and benefits of (right/left) trigeminal nerve block were discussed in detail. The patient understands and accepts that the risks include, but are not limited to, increase in pain, nerve injury, infection, bleeding, hematoma, brain injury, paralysis, stroke, and death. Alternatives to nerve blocks, or noninterventional therapy were discussed, and informed consent obtained.

(*continued*)

(continued)

DESCRIPTION OF PROCEDURE
Intravenous access was established. The patient was escorted to the fluoroscopy suite and placed in the supine position. Noninvasive monitoring was applied. Universal Site and Side Protocol was followed and documented. Safe Injection and Infection Control Practices as recommended by the Center for Disease Control, including the use of face mask, were strictly followed. The face is widely prepped using isopropyl alcohol per protocol, and sterile drapes applied. Time-out was performed. Landmarks of the pterygoid plate were identified. Using a 25-gauge needle, a skin wheal was raised with 1% lidocaine. A 25-gauge 3.5-inch short bevel needle was advanced on the _____ inferior to the pterygoid plate where the trigeminal nerve lies under fluoroscopic guidance. Appropriate needle placement was confirmed using anteroposterior (AP) and lateral views of the fluoroscope. At this point, 2 mL of Omnipaque-240 contrast was injected under live fluoroscopic guidance through a T-Connector extension tubing outlining positive uptake of the trigeminal nerve. After negative aspiration for heme and cerebrospinal fluid (CSF), a total volume of 2 mL of .25% bupivacaine was injected with _____ mg of dexamethasone through the needle. Once the procedure was completed, all needles were withdrawn from the patient intact. A bandage was applied to the puncture site. The patient tolerated this sequence well, there were no complications noted. The patient was discharged home in hemodynamically and neurologically stable condition, with review of postprocedural instructions.

Plan: We will follow up with the patient in 2 to 4 weeks to review the patient's pain diary for consideration of pulsed radiofrequency ablation of the trigeminal nerve.

_____

Attending Physician

Subacromial Bursa Injection

- Indications: Subdeltoid (subacromial) bursitis, shoulder impingement syndrome, adhesive capsulitis (frozen shoulder syndrome), rotator cuff tendinosis

Sample Procedure Note

PREOPERATIVE DIAGNOSIS: Degenerative joint disease
upper extremity
Limb pain upper extremity
Other nerve root plexus
disorder
POSTOPERATIVE DIAGNOSIS: Same
SURGEON: _____
ASSISTANT: _____
TITLE OF PROCEDURE: _____ Subacromial bursa
injection with fluoroscopy
(Video 9.2)

https://bcove.video/2wEm7po

ANESTHESIA: Local anesthesia
ESTIMATED BLOOD LOSS: None
COMPLICATIONS: None

Indications: Patient has been complaining of pain in the _____
shoulder. Our plan is to perform an intra-articular shoulder joint
injection today. The risks and benefits of an intra-articular shoulder
joint injection were discussed in detail. The patient understands
and accepts that the risks include, but are not limited to, increase
in pain, nerve injury, infection, bleeding, hematoma, stroke, and
death. Alternatives to nerve blocks, or noninterventional therapy
were discussed, and informed consent obtained.

DESCRIPTION OF PROCEDURE
The patient was escorted to the fluoroscopy suite and placed
in the seated position. Noninvasive monitoring was applied.
Universal Site and Side Protocol was followed and documented.
Safe Injection and Infection Control Practices as recommended
by the Center for Disease Control were strictly followed.
The _____ shoulder area is widely prepped using isopropyl
alcohol per protocol, and sterile drapes applied. Time-out
was performed. Landmarks of the clavicle, humeral head, and
coracoid process were easily identified. Using a 30-gauge needle,
a skin wheal was raised with 1% lidocaine. A 30-gauge 1.5-
inch short bevel needle was placed into the _____ shoulder

(*continued*)

(*continued*)

> joint using the posterior lateral approach (subacromial) without difficulty. Once the shoulder joint was entered, there was negative aspiration for heme. At this point, 40 mg of Kenalog with _____ mL of .25% preservative-free bupivacaine was injected without complication. Once the procedure was completed, all needles were withdrawn from the patient intact. A bandage was applied to the puncture site. The patient tolerated this procedure well, there were no complications noted. The patient was discharged home in hemodynamically and neurologically stable condition, with review of postprocedural instructions.
>
> **Plan:** We will follow up with the clinic in 2 to 4 weeks.

Trochanteric Bursa Injection

- Indications: Hip pain secondary to inflammation of the trochanteric bursa (trochanteric bursitis)

Sample Procedure Note

PREOPERATIVE DIAGNOSIS:	Trochanteric bursitis
	Hip pain
	Limb pain
POSTOPERATIVE DIAGNOSIS:	Same
SURGEON:	_____
ASSISTANT:	_____
TITLE OF PROCEDURE:	Diagnostic_____
	trochanteric bursa injection
	under fluoroscopic guidance
	Bursa arthrogram
	interpretation under
	fluoroscopy (**Video 9.3**)

https://bcove.video/2wDNTCe

ANESTHESIA:	Local Anesthesia
ESTIMATED BLOOD LOSS:	None
COMPLICATIONS:	None

(*continued*)

Indications: _____ year-old _____ (male/female) complaining of pain in the hip, consistent with trochanteric bursitis. Our plan is to perform a diagnostic trochanteric bursa injection. The risks and benefits of _____ trochanteric bursa injections were discussed in detail. The patient understands and accepts that the risks include, but are not limited to, increase in pain, nerve injury, infection, bleeding, hematoma, paralysis, stroke, and death. Alternatives to nerve blocks, or noninterventional therapy were discussed, and informed consent obtained.

DESCRIPTION OF PROCEDURE
Intravenous access was established. The patient was escorted to the fluoroscopy suite and placed in the supine position. Noninvasive monitoring was applied. Universal Site and Side Protocol was followed and documented. Safe Injection and Infection Control Practices as recommended by the Center for Disease Control, including the use of face mask, were strictly followed. The hip area is widely prepped using isopropyl alcohol per protocol, and sterile drapes applied. Time-out was performed. Landmarks of the femoral head, trochanteric bursa were identified. Using a 25-gauge needle, a skin wheal was raised with 1% lidocaine. A 22-gauge 3.5-inch curved Quincke spinal needle was advanced on the _____ trochanteric bursa under fluoroscopic guidance. Once the trochanteric bursa was in contact, AP and lateral views of the fluoroscope confirmed adequate needle placement. At this point, 2 mL of Omnipaque-240 contrast was injected under live fluoroscopic guidance through a T-Connector extension tubing outlining positive uptake of the trochanteric bursa. After negative aspiration for heme, a total volume of 8 mL of .25% bupivacaine was injected with 40 mg of Kenalog through the needle. Once the procedure was completed, all needles were withdrawn from the patient intact. A bandage was applied to the puncture site. The patient tolerated this sequence well, there were no complications noted. The patient was discharged home in hemodynamically and neurologically stable condition, with review of postprocedural instructions.

Plan: We will follow up with the patient in 2 to 4 weeks.

Piriformis Injection
- Indications: Piriformis syndrome

Sample Procedure Note

PREOPERATIVE DIAGNOSIS: Piriformis syndrome
Low back pain
POSTOPERATIVE DIAGNOSIS: Same
SURGEON: _____
ASSISTANT: _____
TITLE OF PROCEDURE: Diagnostic _____ piriformis
injection under fluoroscopic
guidance (**Video 9.4**)

https://bcove.video/2rHi1HW

ANESTHESIA: Monitored anesthesia care
ESTIMATED BLOOD LOSS: None
COMPLICATIONS: None

Indications: _____ year-old _____ (male/female) complaining of low back and lower extremity pain, consistent with piriformis syndrome. Our plan is to perform a diagnostic piriformis injection under fluoroscopic guidance today. The risks and benefits of _____ piriformis injection were discussed in detail. The patient understands and accepts that the risks include, but are not limited to, increase in pain, nerve injury, infection, bleeding, hematoma, paralysis, spinal headache, stroke, discitis, and death. Alternatives to nerve blocks, or noninterventional therapy were discussed, and informed consent obtained.

DESCRIPTION OF PROCEDURE
Intravenous access was established. The patient was escorted to the fluoroscopy suite and placed in the prone position. Noninvasive monitoring was applied. Universal Site and Side Protocol was followed and documented. Safe Injection and Infection Control Practices as recommended by the Center for Disease Control, including the use of face mask, were strictly followed. The low back and buttock area is widely prepped using isopropyl alcohol per protocol, and sterile drapes applied. Time-out was performed. Using fluoroscopic guidance, the sacrum, femoral head, and pubic symphysis were identified. Using a 25-gauge needle, a skin wheal was raised with 1% lidocaine. Under fluoroscopic guidance in the AP and lateral views, a 22-gauge 3.5-inch curved Quincke tip spinal needle was advanced to near the femoral head and pelvis where the piriformis muscle lies on the _____. AP and lateral projections

(continued)

(continued)

of the fluoroscope confirmed adequate needle placement. Needle placement was then confirmed using 2 mL of Omnipaque-240 contrast outlining a myogram. There was no evidence of intrathecal, epidural, or intravascular spread. After negative aspiration for heme and CSF, a total volume of 8 mL of .25% bupivacaine was injected with 40 mg of Kenalog through the needle. Once the procedure was completed, all needles were withdrawn from the patient intact. A bandage was applied to the puncture site. The patient tolerated this sequence well, there were no complications noted. The patient was discharged home in hemodynamically and neurologically stable condition, with review of postprocedural instructions.

Plan: We will follow up with the patient in 2 to 4 weeks.

_____

Attending Physician

Genicular Nerve Block
- Indications: Patients with chronic knee pain secondary to osteoarthritis, patients with failed knee replacement, patients who are unable to undergo knee replacement, and patients who want to avoid knee replacement surgery

Sample Procedure Note

PREOPERATIVE DIAGNOSIS:	Osteoarthritis Limb pain Other nerve root plexus disorder
POSTOPERATIVE DIAGNOSIS:	Same
SURGEON:	_____
ASSISTANT:	_____
TITLE OF PROCEDURE:	Diagnostic _____ genicular nerve block under fluoroscopic guidance (**Video 9.5**)
https://bcove.video/2IEbqI9	
ANESTHESIA:	Monitored anesthesia care
ESTIMATED BLOOD LOSS:	None
COMPLICATIONS	None

(continued)

(continued)

Indications: _____ year-old (male/female) complaining of pain in the knee, consistent with osteoarthritis. Our plan is to perform a diagnostic genicular nerve block. The risks and benefits of _____ genicular nerve block were discussed in detail. The patient understands and accepts that the risks include, but are not limited to, increase in pain, nerve injury, infection, bleeding, and hematoma. Alternatives to nerve blocks, or noninterventional therapy were discussed, and informed consent obtained.

DESCRIPTION OF PROCEDURE
Intravenous access was established. The patient was escorted to the fluoroscopy suite and placed in the supine position with a pillow behind the popliteal fossa. Noninvasive monitoring was applied. Universal Site and Side Protocol was followed and documented. Safe Injection and Infection Control Practices as recommended by the Center for Disease Control, including the use of face mask, were strictly followed. The knee area is widely prepped using isopropyl alcohol per protocol, and sterile drapes applied. Time-out was performed. Landmarks of the patella, medial and lateral epicondyle were identified. Using a 25-gauge needle, a skin wheal was raised with 1% lidocaine. A 22-gauge 3.5-inch curved Quincke tip spinal needle was advanced over the medial and lateral femoral condyle and over the medial tibial condyle until bone was contacted on the _____ where the medial, lateral, and inferomedial genicular nerve lies. After negative aspiration for heme, 2 mL of Omnipaque-240 was injected through a T-Connector extension tubing under real-time fluoroscopy outlining a neurogram. At this point, a total volume of 3 mL of .75% bupivacaine was injected with 40 mg of Kenalog in divided doses. Once the procedure was completed, all needles were withdrawn from the patient intact. A bandage was applied to the puncture site. The patient tolerated this sequence well, there were no complications noted. The patient was discharged home in hemodynamically and neurologically stable condition, with review of postprocedural instructions. We will follow up with the patient in 2 to 4 weeks.

Plan: If the patient receives 50% or greater pain relief from the procedure, we will perform radiofrequency thermal coagulation of the genicular nerves under fluoroscopic guidance.

_____
Attending Physician

List of Videos

Video 9.1 Trigeminal Nerve Block

https://bcove.video/2jTZcwU

Video 9.2 Subacromial Bursa Injection

https://bcove.video/2wEm7po

Video 9.3 Trochanteric Bursa Injection

https://bcove.video/2wDNTCe

Video 9.4 Piriformis Injection

https://bcove.video/2rHi1HW

Video 9.5 Genicular Nerve Block

https://bcove.video/2IEbqI9

ICD-9 DIAGNOSIS CODE	ICD-9 DIAGNOSIS DESCRIPTION	ICD-10 DIAGNOSIS CODE	ICD-10 DIAGNOSIS DESCRIPTION
338.4	Chronic pain syndrome	G894	Chronic pain syndrome
350.1	Trigeminal neuralgia	G500	Trigeminal neuralgia
353.6	Phantom limb pain	G546	Phantom limb syndrome with pain
354.0	Carpal tunnel syndrome	G5600	Carpal tunnel syndrome, unspecified upper limb
		G5601	Carpal tunnel syndrome, right upper limb
		G5602	Carpal tunnel syndrome, left upper limb
354.2	Ulnar neuropathy	G5620	Lesion of ulnar nerve, unspecified upper limb
		G5621	Lesion of ulnar nerve, right upper limb
		G5622	Lesion of ulnar nerve, left upper limb

(continued)

(continued)

ICD-9 DIAGNOSIS CODE	ICD-9 DIAGNOSIS DESCRIPTION	ICD-10 DIAGNOSIS CODE	ICD-10 DIAGNOSIS DESCRIPTION
355.5	Tarsal tunnel syndrome	G5750	Tarsal tunnel syndrome, unspecified lower limb
		G5751	Tarsal tunnel syndrome, right lower limb
		G5752	Tarsal tunnel syndrome, left lower limb
355.9	Piriformis syndrome	G588	Other specified mononeuropathies
		G589	Mononeuropathy, unspecified
		G59	Mononeuropathy in diseases classified elsewhere
356.9	Peripheral neuropathy	G609	Hereditary and idiopathic neuropathy, unspecified
524.60	Temporomandibular joint dysfunction	M2660	Temporomandibular joint disorder, unspecified
715.15	Osteoarthritis, shoulder	M19011	Primary osteoarthritis, right shoulder
		M19012	Primary osteoarthritis, left shoulder

(continued)

(*continued*)

		M19019	Primary osteoarthritis, unspecified shoulder
715.16	Osteoarthritis, knee	M1710	Unilateral primary osteoarthritis, unspecified knee
		M1711	Unilateral primary osteoarthritis, right knee
		M1712	Unilateral primary osteoarthritis, left knee
721.0	Cervical spondylosis without myelopathy	M4721	Other spondylosis with radiculopathy, occipito–atlanto–axial region
		M4722	Other spondylosis with radiculopathy, cervical region
		M4723	Other spondylosis with radiculopathy, cervicothoracic region
		M47811	Spondylosis without myelopathy or radiculopathy, occipito–atlanto–axial region

(*continued*)

(*continued*)

ICD-9 DIAGNOSIS CODE	ICD-9 DIAGNOSIS DESCRIPTION	ICD-10 DIAGNOSIS CODE	ICD-10 DIAGNOSIS DESCRIPTION
		M47812	Spondylosis without myelopathy or radiculopathy, cervical region
		M47813	Spondylosis without myelopathy or radiculopathy, cervicothoracic region
		M47891	Other spondylosis, occipito–atlanto–axial region
		M47892	Other spondylosis, cervical region
		M47893	Other spondylosis, cervicothoracic region
721.3	Lumbar spondylosis without myelopathy	M4726	Other spondylosis with radiculopathy, lumbar region
		M4727	Other spondylosis with radiculopathy, lumbosacral region

(*continued*)

(*continued*)

		M4728	Other spondylosis with radiculopathy, sacral and sacrococcygeal region
		M47816	Spondylosis without myelopathy or radiculopathy, lumbar region
		M47817	Spondylosis without myelopathy or radiculopathy, lumbosacral region
		M47818	Spondylosis without myelopathy or radiculopathy, sacral and sacrococcygeal region
		M47896	Other spondylosis, lumbar region
		M47897	Other spondylosis, lumbosacral region

(*continued*)

(*continued*)

ICD-9 DIAGNOSIS CODE	ICD-9 DIAGNOSIS DESCRIPTION	ICD-10 DIAGNOSIS CODE	ICD-10 DIAGNOSIS DESCRIPTION
		M47898	Other spondylosis, sacral and sacrococcygeal region
722.0	Cervical herniated disc without myelopathy	M5020	Other cervical disc displacement, unspecified cervical region
		M5021	Other cervical disc displacement, high cervical region
		M5022	Other cervical disc displacement, midcervical region
		M5023	Other cervical disc displacement, cervicothoracic region
722.10	Lumbar herniated disc	M5126	Other intervertebral disc displacement, lumbar region
		M5127	Other intervertebral disc displacement, lumbosacral region

(*continued*)

(continued)

722.4	Cervical degenerative disc disease	M5030	Other cervical disc degeneration, unspecified cervical region
		M5031	Other cervical disc degeneration, high cervical region
		M5032	Other cervical disc degeneration, midcervical region
722.4	Cervical degenerative disc disease	M5033	Other cervical disc degeneration, cervicothoracic region
722.52	Lumbosacral degenerated disc disease	M5136	Other intervertebral disc degeneration, lumbar region
		M5137	Other intervertebral disc degeneration, lumbosacral region

(continued)

(continued)

ICD-9 DIAGNOSIS CODE	ICD-9 DIAGNOSIS DESCRIPTION	ICD-10 DIAGNOSIS CODE	ICD-10 DIAGNOSIS DESCRIPTION
722.83	Lumbar failed back surgery syndrome	M96.1	Postlaminectomy syndrome, not elsewhere classified
723.0	Cervical spinal stenosis	M4801	Spinal stenosis, occipito–atlanto–axial region
		M4802	Spinal stenosis, cervical region
		M4803	Spinal stenosis, cervicothoracic region
		M9920	Subluxation stenosis of neural canal of head region
		M9921	Subluxation stenosis of neural canal of cervical region
		M9930	Osseous stenosis of neural canal of head region
		M9931	Osseous stenosis of neural canal of cervical region
		M9940	Connective tissue stenosis of neural canal of head region

(continued)

(continued)

		M99.41	Connective tissue stenosis of neural canal of cervical region
		M99.50	Intervertebral disc stenosis of neural canal of head region
		M99.51	Intervertebral disc stenosis of neural canal of cervical region
		M99.60	Osseous and subluxation stenosis of intervertebral foramina of head region
		M99.61	Osseous and subluxation stenosis of intervertebral foramina of cervical region
		M99.70	Connective tissue and disc stenosis of intervertebral foramina of head region

(continued)

(*continued*)

ICD-9 DIAGNOSIS CODE	ICD-9 DIAGNOSIS DESCRIPTION	ICD-10 DIAGNOSIS CODE	ICD-10 DIAGNOSIS DESCRIPTION
		M99.71	Connective tissue and disc stenosis of intervertebral foramina of cervical region
723.1	Cervicalgia (neck pain)	M54.2	Cervicalgia
723.4	Cervical radiculopathy (radiculitis)	M50.10	Cervical disc disorder with radiculopathy, unspecified cervical region
		M50.11	Cervical disc disorder with radiculopathy, high cervical region
		M50.12	Cervical disc disorder with radiculopathy, midcervical region
		M50.13	Cervical disc disorder with radiculopathy, cervicothoracic region
723.8	Occipital neuralgia/ headache	M54.11	Radiculopathy, occipito–atlanto– axial region
		M54.12	Radiculopathy, cervical region

(*continued*)

(continued)

		M54.13	Radiculopathy, cervicothoracic region
		M53.81	Other specified dorsopathies, occipito–atlanto–axial region
		M53.82	Other specified dorsopathies, cervical region
		M53.83	Other specified dorsopathies, cervicothoracic region
		M54.81	Occipital neuralgia
724.02	Spinal stenosis of lumbar region	M48.06	Spinal stenosis, lumbar region
		M48.07	Spinal stenosis, lumbosacral region
		M99.23	Subluxation stenosis of neural canal of lumbar region
		M99.33	Osseous stenosis of neural canal of lumbar region
		M99.43	Connective tissue stenosis of neural canal of lumbar region

(continued)

(continued)

ICD-9 DIAGNOSIS CODE	ICD-9 DIAGNOSIS DESCRIPTION	ICD-10 DIAGNOSIS CODE	ICD-10 DIAGNOSIS DESCRIPTION
724.02	Spinal stenosis of lumbar region	N99.53	Intervertebral disc stenosis of neural canal of lumbar region
		N99.63	Osseous and subluxation stenosis of intervertebral foramina of lumbar region
		N99.73	Connective tissue and disc stenosis of intervertebral foramina of lumbar region
724.2	Low back pain (lumbago)	M54.5	Low back pain
724.3	Sciatica	M54.30	Sciatica, unspecified side
		M54.31	Sciatica, right side
		M54.32	Sciatica, left side
		M54.40	Lumbago with sciatica, unspecified side
		M54.41	Lumbago with sciatica, right side
		M54.42	Lumbago with sciatica, left side

(continued)

(*continued*)

724.4	Thoracic/lumbosacral neuritis/radiculitis, unspecified	M51.14	Intervertebral disc disorders with radiculopathy, thoracic region
		M51.15	Intervertebral disc disorders with radiculopathy, thoracolumbar region
		M51.16	Intervertebral disc disorders with radiculopathy, lumbar region
		M51.17	Intervertebral disc disorders with radiculopathy, lumbosacral region
		M54.14	Radiculopathy, thoracic region
		M54.15	Radiculopathy, thoracolumbar region
		M54.16	Radiculopathy, lumbar region
		M54.17	Radiculopathy, lumbosacral region

(*continued*)

(continued)

ICD-9 DIAGNOSIS CODE	ICD-9 DIAGNOSIS DESCRIPTION	ICD-10 DIAGNOSIS CODE	ICD-10 DIAGNOSIS DESCRIPTION
724.6	Disorders of the sacrum	M43.27	Fusion of spine, lumbosacral region
		M43.28	Fusion of spine, sacral and sacrococcygeal region
		M53.2X7	Spinal instabilities, lumbosacral region
		M53.2X8	Spinal instabilities, sacral and sacrococcygeal region
		M53.3	Sacrococcygeal disorders, not elsewhere classified
		M53.86	Other specified dorsopathies, lumbar region
		M53.87	Other specified dorsopathies, lumbosacral region
		M53.88	Other specified dorsopathies, sacral and sacrococcygeal region

(continued)

(continued)

726.0	Adhesive capsulitis	M75.00	Adhesive capsulitis of unspecified shoulder
		M75.01	Adhesive capsulitis of right shoulder
		M75.02	Adhesive capsulitis of left shoulder
726.10	Subacromial bursitis	M66.211	Spontaneous rupture of extensor tendons, right shoulder
		M66.212	Spontaneous rupture of extensor tendons, left shoulder
		M66.219	Spontaneous rupture of extensor tendons, unspecified shoulder
		M66.811	Spontaneous rupture of other tendons, right shoulder

(continued)

(*continued*)

ICD-9 DIAGNOSIS CODE	ICD-9 DIAGNOSIS DESCRIPTION	ICD-10 DIAGNOSIS CODE	ICD-10 DIAGNOSIS DESCRIPTION
		M66.812	Spontaneous rupture of other tendons, left shoulder
		M66.819	Spontaneous rupture of other tendons, unspecified shoulder
726.10	Subacromial bursitis	M75.50	Bursitis of unspecified shoulder
		M75.51	Bursitis of right shoulder
		M75.52	Bursitis of left shoulder
726.32	Lateral epicondylitis	M77.10	Lateral epicondylitis, unspecified elbow
		M77.11	Lateral epicondylitis, right elbow
		M77.12	Lateral epicondylitis, left elbow
726.5	Trochanteric bursitis	M25.751	Osteophyte, right hip
		M25.752	Osteophyte, left hip
		M25.759	Osteophyte, unspecified hip

(*continued*)

(*continued*)

		M70.60	Trochanteric bursitis, unspecified hip
		M70.61	Trochanteric bursitis, right hip
		M70.62	Trochanteric bursitis, left hip
		M70.70	Other bursitis of hip, unspecified hip
		M70.71	Other bursitis of hip, right hip
		M70.72	Other bursitis of hip, left hip
		M76.30	Iliotibial band syndrome, unspecified leg
		M76.31	Iliotibial band syndrome, right leg
		M76.32	Iliotibial band syndrome, left leg
728.71	Plantar fasciitis	M72.2	Plantar fascial fibromatosis
728.87	Muscle weakness (generalized)	M62.81	Muscle weakness (generalized)
729.1	Myofascial pain/ fibromyalgia	M60.80	Other myositis, unspecified site

(*continued*)

(continued)

ICD-9 DIAGNOSIS CODE	ICD-9 DIAGNOSIS DESCRIPTION	ICD-10 DIAGNOSIS CODE	ICD-10 DIAGNOSIS DESCRIPTION
729.1	Myofascial pain/ fibromyalgia	M79.1	Myalgia
		M79.7	Fibromyalgia
738.4	Spondylolisthesis	M43.00	Spondylolysis, site unspecified
		M43.01	Spondylolysis, occipito–atlanto– axial region
		M43.02	Spondylolysis, cervical region
		M43.03	Spondylolysis, cervicothoracic region
		M43.04	Spondylolysis, thoracic region
		M43.05	Spondylolysis, thoracolumbar region
		M43.06	Spondylolysis, lumbar region
		M43.07	Spondylolysis, lumbosacral region
		M43.08	Spondylolysis, sacral and sacrococcygeal region

(continued)

(*continued*)

		M43.09	Spondylolysis, multiple sites in spine
		M43.10	Spondylolisthesis, site unspecified
		M43.11	Spondylolisthesis, occipito–atlanto–axial region
		M43.12	Spondylolisthesis, cervical region
		M43.13	Spondylolisthesis, cervicothoracic region
		M43.14	Spondylolisthesis, thoracic region
		M43.15	Spondylolisthesis, thoracolumbar region
		M43.16	Spondylolisthesis, lumbar region
		M43.17	Spondylolisthesis, lumbosacral region
738.4	Spondylolisthesis	M43.18	Spondylolisthesis, sacral and sacrococcygeal region
		M43.19	Spondylolisthesis, multiple sites in spine

(*continued*)

(*continued*)

ICD-9 DIAGNOSIS CODE	ICD-9 DIAGNOSIS DESCRIPTION	ICD-10 DIAGNOSIS CODE	ICD-10 DIAGNOSIS DESCRIPTION
847.0	Cervical sprain/strain	S13.4XXA	Sprain of ligaments of cervical spine, initial encounter
		S13.8XXA	Sprain of joints and ligaments of other parts of neck, initial encounter
		S16.1XXA	Strain of muscle, fascia and tendon at neck level, initial encounter
847.1	Thoracic sprain	S23.3XXA	Sprain of ligaments of thoracic spine, initial encounter
		S23.8XXA	Sprain of other specified parts of thorax, initial encounter
847.2	Lumbar sprain	S33.5XXA	Sprain of ligaments of lumbar spine, initial encounter
Postlaminectomy syndrome (FBSS)		M96.1	
Intercostal neuralgia		G58.0	

FBSS, failed back surgery syndrome; ICD, International Classification of Diseases.

Index